ABOUT THE AUTHOR

William J. (Jody) Wilkinson, M.D., M.S., is a physician and exercise physiologist at the Cooper Institute in Dallas, Texas. He did his medical training at the University of Texas Health Science Center in San Antonio, Texas, and Baylor University Medical Center in Dallas. Dr. Wilkinson is the Director of The Cooper Institute Weight Management Research Center. He strongly believes in using biblical teaching to motivate people to take care of their physical bodies and enjoy abundant living. Jody and his wife, Natalie, have been married 10 years and have two daughters, Jordan and Sarah, and twin sons, Joel and Cooper.

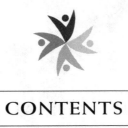

CONTENTS

health4life

JODY WILKINSON, M.D.

From Gospel Light
Ventura, California, U.S.A.

Regal Books is a ministry of Gospel Light, a Christian publisher dedicated to serving the local church. We believe God's vision for Gospel Light is to provide church leaders with biblical, user-friendly materials that will help them evangelize, disciple and minister to children, youth and families.

It is our prayer that this Regal book will help you discover biblical truth for your own life and help you minister to others. May God richly bless you.

For a free catalog of resources from Regal Books/Gospel Light, please call your Christian supplier or contact us at 1-800-4-GOSPEL *or* www.regalbooks.com.

PUBLISHING STAFF
William T. Greig, Chairman
Kyle Duncan, Publisher
Dr. Elmer L. Towns, Senior Consulting Publisher
Pam Weston, Senior Editor
Patti Pennington Virtue, Associate Editor
Jeff Kempton, Editorial Assistant
Hilary Young, Editorial Assistant
Bayard Taylor, M.Div., Senior Editor, Biblical and Theological Issues
Samantha A. Hsu, Cover and Internal Designer

CAUTION
The information contained in this book is intended to be solely informational and educational. It is assumed that the First Place participant will consult a medical or health professional before beginning this or any other weight-loss or physical-fitness program.

Physical Well-Being

Nutrition

Planning for Good Nutrition

An Ounce of Prevention

FOREWORD

If I had to say just one thing I love most about the First Place program, it would be that First Place ministers to the total person, not just the physical side that the world thinks is most important. First Samuel 16:7 says, "The LORD does not look at the things man looks at. Man looks at the outward appearance, but the LORD looks at the heart." *Health 4 Life* speaks to each of us in every area of our lives: emotional, spiritual, mental and physical. Learning what it means to live a life of balance in all of these areas allows us to walk in freedom and victory every day.

The last five years of my life have been personally challenging. My husband was diagnosed with stage four cancer in October 1997. We lost our precious 39-year-old daughter Shari in November of 2001 when she was struck and killed by an 18-year-old girl who made the decision to drink and drive. We have also had the challenge of caring for my aging mom and having her live with us for two and a half years. Because of the lessons I have learned about balance in First Place, I am able not only to cope but also to experience joy and victory that is hard for this lost world to comprehend or understand.

Our heavenly Father has a purpose and plan for our lives. As Jesus stated, "I have come that they may have life, and have it to the full" (John 10:10). The purpose of *Health 4 Life* is to give you information that will help and guide you to establish a balanced lifestyle.

God wants us to be well emotionally. He desires for us to win over stress and worry. He challenges us daily to change who we are by changing what we put into our minds and changing how we think. Scripture memory is the most important tool to accomplish emotional health. Thousands of First Place members have memorized Scripture verses and have found emotional healing through God's Word.

God wants us to be well spiritually. Learning how to have a daily quiet time is essential to spiritual wellness. Bible study and the daily reading of Scripture will bring about the balanced life each of us desperately desires. *Health 4 Life* gives definite instruction in the spiritual area.

God wants us to be well mentally. Many of us aspire to being mentally whole, but we need the tools to help us get there. *Health 4 Life* provides practical help and training for sound thinking and sound living. One of the greatest helps I have received from my First Place walk is learning that each of us is given the same 24 hours every day. Learning how to manage my time well has brought the mental wholeness I desired.

God wants us to be well physically. Dr. Jody Wilkinson has devoted his life to helping others find wellness in every area. A lifetime of research has gone into the physical information in *Health 4 Life*. The material contained in this section—when applied—becomes the foundation for developing a healthy lifestyle, not only for ourselves, but for all those we love.

You're in for the greatest experience of your life—learning to live a life of balance will bring true joy.

Carole Lewis
National Director of First Place

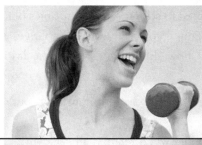

emotional

WELL-
BEING

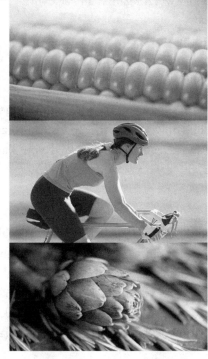

the challenge to change

Change is never easy. In fact, most people successful in changing a lifestyle habit make several attempts before reaching their goal. Studies reveal that people who have successfully quit smoking attempted to stop three to four times before achieving their goal. The key is to keep trying; if you really want to change, you can do it. The following statistics reveal how difficult it is to make lasting changes in lifestyle habits:

- Over 50 percent of people who start an exercise program drop out within the first three to six months.
- More than 80 percent of people who lose weight gain it all back within three to five years.
- Less than 30 percent of people who make a New Year's resolution stick with it to the end of the year.
- Only 30 percent of people who attempt to stop smoking are successful.

The keys to successful lifestyle change are staying on track when times get tough and bouncing back after a setback. The only way to succeed is to realize that you will be tempted and experience setbacks along the way. If you plan ahead and have realistic expectations, you will reach your goals.

Overcoming Temptation

Have you ever been working toward a goal or maybe even achieved your goal, only to have something come along and knock you off course and put you right back where you started? When making lifestyle changes, such as losing weight or starting an exercise program, people report several situations or factors that often knock them off track. It's important to understand what things will make it difficult for you to achieve your goals. Do any of the following sound familiar to you?

- Stress and other emotional factors
- Illness or injury (to self or a loved one)
- Holidays and special occasions
- The influence of others
- Overwork
- Bad weather
- Travel and vacations

Once you understand how you're likely to be tempted and where your challenges are going to come from, you can begin building a plan that won't allow these situations to knock you off course. Don't let temptation, challenges and setbacks keep you from achieving your goals. When it comes to your health, happiness and quality of life, don't let anything come between you and your goals. Don't let guilt, negative thinking, embarrassment, feelings of failure, temporary setbacks or anything else come between you and a worthwhile goal. For encouragement, read Romans 8:28-39. The choice is up to you: You can view setbacks and slipups as failures, or you can view them as learning opportunities to help you grow stronger.

When it comes to making lifestyle changes, you *will* be tempted. Read the account of the temptation of Eve in Genesis 3:1-6. Look at many of the ways in which she was tempted.

- "You will not surely die . . . you will be like God" (spiritual)
- "The woman saw that the fruit of the tree was pleasing" (emotional)
- "Desirable for gaining wisdom" (intellectual)
- "She took some and ate it" (physical)
- "She also gave some to her husband" (social)

Don't get discouraged when you are tempted. God will provide you with a way out (see 1 Corinthians 10:13). If you look for the way out and are willing to act on what God provides, you can overcome temptation. One of the best ways to overcome temptation is to rely on God's Word (see Psalm 119:11; Matthew 4:1-11). Build a list of memory verses that can help you through temptation and difficult times.

A Lesson on Learning

When making lifestyle changes, it's important to learn from both your successes and your setbacks. If you have set a worthwhile goal, it's important to do all you can to achieve success. When you are tempted or you experience a setback, think about what went wrong. Explore ways you can prevent it from happening next time. Ask yourself if your expectations and feelings are realistic. Most importantly, avoid negative thinking.

letting others help you succeed

It's important to find people who can help you achieve and maintain your goals and then get them involved in providing the support and encouragement you need. Communication is the cornerstone of any relationship. You must tell your partner what you need. Ask him or her to do specific things to help you. Never expect your partner to read your mind. Tell him or her when you need encouragement. Point out—in a positive way—when you need him or her to respond or treat you differently. Ask frequently what you can do for your partner. Surprise him or her with rewards that show your appreciation. For a partnership to be successful, the relationship must be one in which each partner gives a little and takes a little.

Kinds of Support

There are many types of support. Think about the types of support you need and who can best help.

- **Do you need someone to talk to?** It's important to be able to share your feelings and experiences with others. Sometimes all you need is someone to listen. It's important to be able to share both positive and negative aspects of your life. With whom can you best share your feelings and experiences?
- **Do you need someone to participate with you?** It's often easier and more fun to make lifestyle changes when others are involved. Would your spouse or a friend go through the program with you? Who would be someone to exercise with? Will it help if your family makes some changes with you?
- **Do you need someone to provide you with encouragement?** It's easier to make changes when others are encouraging and supporting you. It's easy to get discouraged when you slip up or don't reach your goals as quickly as you would like. Who can help pick you up when you get down and discouraged? Who is a good encourager for you?

    Sometimes it's important to have constructive criticism. Who would help you stay on your goals and push you when you need it?

    Ask others to give you the feedback you need—and be willing to accept what they say. Who is the best person to help you in this way?

- **Do you need someone to help with other aspects of your life?** Changing your lifestyle takes time and effort. Do you need help with personal responsibilities, so you can free up time to work out, attend a group meeting or cook a healthy meal? Who can help you around the house or at work so that you will have more time to make the changes you need?

Keys to a Successful Partnership

- **First you must set realistic goals.** Let family and friends know how important making a particular change is to you. Let them know you are committed to success.
- **When asking for help, be as specific as you can.** Tell others exactly how they can help you. Better yet, work out a plan together and develop a contract.
- **Communicate openly and often about your thoughts, feelings and needs.** Practice positive communication—avoid being negative or critical.
- **Never expect one person to be all things for you.**
- **Be sensitive to the needs of others.** Always consider how you can help those who help you. Don't hesitate to ask for the help you need, but try to offer something in return. Reward others for their help: say thank you, buy them small gifts or treat them to special occasions.

overcoming difficult situations

A prudent man foresees difficulty and plans accordingly.
(See Proverbs 27:12.)

Difficult situations, temptations and setbacks are an expected and natural part of making lifestyle changes. Many people envision weight loss as a race that begins with a mad dash down the track and finishes at the line in record time. It's important to know that the road to change has many hurdles and hazards along the way—and it's a lifelong journey! It's important to know your course, set your eye on the prize and run with endurance the race set before you (see Philippians 3:12-14; Hebrews 12:1).

Review the following three-step process to help you understand how and when you will be tempted. Most important, use it to develop a plan of attack when temptation strikes or you experience a setback.

Step 1—Identify Difficult Situations

The first step is to know your course and what lies ahead. Start by identifying situations—people, places, feelings and foods—that make it difficult for you to stick with your plan. Think carefully about your behavior. Do you eat when you are lonely or angry or when you feel out of control in other areas of your life? Do you tend to overeat at parties or other social situations? Is there a certain restaurant where you almost always overeat? Talk to family and friends to get a better understanding of those situations that are difficult for you.

Step 2—Understand Your Usual Response

Perhaps the most crucial part of any plan is understanding how you respond to difficult situations and slipups. Ingrain this in your mind: *Temptation and slipups are an important part of the process of change.* Temptation and slipups are not failures; they're opportunities to learn and move closer to your goal. Unfortunately, because of negative thinking or unrealistic expectations, many people allow a slipup to throw them completely off course. By knowing and understanding your usual responses, you can turn what you think is weakness into strength. How do you usually respond when faced with a difficult situation? Do you often give in to temptation or the influence of others? Do you feel guilty when you make mistakes? Do you feel like a failure? Have slipups knocked you off your program in the past?

Step 3—Develop a Plan of Action

After identifying difficult situations and how you typically respond, you can begin to plan a solid defense. A prudent person foresees difficulty and plans accordingly. Having a plan provides you with a road map that will help you stay on course. Make a list of strategies you can use to get you through difficult situations. For example, how can you turn negative thoughts—*Now that I've blown it, what's the use of trying?*—into more positive responses—*What went wrong here? How can I avoid this next time?* Don't forget the importance of enlisting support. Friends and family are a great source of help and encouragement—use them!

- Ask your spouse to drop off or pick up the children so you can work out.
- Give your friends a list of restaurants that make it easy for you to stick to your eating plan.
- Find someone to walk with you during your lunch break.
- Find an accountability partner to check in with once a week.

Make a list of situations that are difficult for you and how you usually respond to them. Begin thinking of ways to respond differently the next time you face a similar situation. What things can you do to help you stay on track?

Keep Your Eyes on the Prize

Remember your goals. Take time to understand yourself and what circumstances make it difficult for you to reach and maintain your goals. Most people are in such a hurry to reach their goals that they fail to plan for difficult situations. People who are successful in making lifestyle changes recognize that setbacks are normal and they make plans for overcoming difficult situations. Also they don't see setbacks as failures but as opportunities. It's what we do over weeks and months that makes the difference in our health and quality of life. If you slip up one day, the next day just pick right up where you left off.

It's also important to reward yourself and feel good about the progress you're making along the way. Recognize and celebrate your success. Lifestyle change and healthier habits bring real benefits. Personal rewards such as feeling better, more energy, better self-esteem and improved health are the strongest motivators. You're more likely to stick with your program if it makes you feel good. You can reward yourself in other ways too. A new outfit, a night out on the town or a weekend getaway are also ways you can reward yourself. Contract with a loved one or friend for special rewards along the way. In this whole process of change, remember who is on your side.

If the LORD delights in a man's way, he makes his steps firm; though he stumble, he will not fall, for the LORD upholds him with his hand.
Psalm 37:23-24

overcoming stress

Do you ever feel like the treadmill of life is stuck on high speed and there's no one around to slow it down? Are the pressures of work, home, finances and other responsibilities piling up so fast, you often wonder if you can keep up? Do you feel like you're being pushed and pulled in so many different directions that you think you might break in two? Do you feel like there's just no time for *you*? Are you having a hard time experiencing the abundant life that Christ desires for you (see John 10:10)? If you identify with *any* of these questions, you're probably stressed.

What Is Stress?

Stress is the response of our bodies or minds to physical or emotional strain, such as overwork or too much worry. Stress or worry occurs when you take your focus off that which is truly important. Some experts refer to stress as "hurry sickness."

Fortunately, God has given us the ability to recognize and respond to challenges. The stress response protects us and allows us to persevere against the Goliaths of life. The body responds to challenges by releasing a number of hormones, such as adrenaline, which rev up the body and prepare it for action. Stress experts refer to this response as "fight or flight." David had a choice whether to fight or run from Goliath. Unfortunately, many of our battles pile up faster than we can keep up, and it's much harder to run from deadlines, traffic jams and bills. In fact, much of our stress is caused by thinking about things that haven't yet happened—and probably never will. Over time, the stress response begins to take its toll on the body, mind and spirit.

The Harmful Effects of Stress

Our bodies are clearly not designed for chronic stress. Stress is linked to heart disease, high blood pressure, obesity, depression and unhealthy habits. Stress causes headaches, backaches and digestive problems. Chronic stress suppresses the immune system and makes the body susceptible to a variety of illnesses. Stress can make you feel angry, irritable, afraid, excited or helpless. Stress makes it hard to sleep or relax, and it leaves you feeling fatigued. It's no wonder that God's Word repeatedly tells us not to worry or be anxious (see Matthew 6:25; John 14:27; Philippians 4:6-7).

To find out if you are stressed, answer each of the following questions:

- Do you often feel tense, nervous or anxious?
- Do you have a hard time relaxing or turning off your thoughts?
- Do you often worry about all the things you have to do?
- Do you have a hard time concentrating or staying focused?
- Do you often feel like things are out of your control?
- Do you constantly feel like you're in a hurry?
- Do you notice that you're irritable or get angry often?
- Do you often take on more than you can handle?

If you answered yes to one or more of these questions, chances are that stress is taking its toll on your health and quality of life. Are you ready to learn some ways to change your response to the challenges of your life?

A Biblical Plan for Taming the Stress Response

Trust in God

> Trust in the LORD with all your heart and lean not on your own understanding;
> in all your ways acknowledge him, and he will make your paths straight.
> Proverbs 3:5-6

Do you view life from God's perspective? Have you gotten out of touch with God and His purpose for your life? Whose strength do you rely on when you're faced with a challenge or feeling overwhelmed? Stress is a signal to return your focus to God. When you're feeling stressed, remember that God loves you and is in control of all things.

Overcome Stress Through Prayer

> Do not be anxious about anything, but in everything, by prayer and petition, with
> thanksgiving, present your requests to God. And the peace of God, which transcends
> all understanding, will guard your hearts and your minds in Christ Jesus.
> Philippians 4:6-7

What happens to your prayer life during times of stress? Never underestimate the power of prayer in dealing with the challenges of life. Learn to trust the Lord; He will provide a way out for you.

Focus on What Is Most Important

Finally, brothers, whatever is true, whatever is noble, whatever is right, whatever is pure, whatever is lovely, whatever is admirable—if anything is excellent or praiseworthy—think about such things. Philippians 4:8

In times of stress, ask yourself if your mind is set on the truth. Are you realistically evaluating and responding to your situation? Are you applying your mind to positive solutions?

Take Positive Steps to Change the Situation

Whatever you have learned or received or heard from me, or seen in me— put it into practice. And the God of peace will be with you. Philippians 4:9

The key to dealing with stress is to take positive action. Nothing is ever changed by worry. Identify the source of your stress and begin taking steps to either eliminate it or deal with it in positive ways.

winning over worry

Who of you by worrying can add a single hour to his life?

Matthew 6:27

Does worry ever interfere with the quality of your life? Does it sometimes make it difficult for you to experience the *abundant* life that Christ desires for you? Are daily responsibilities such as work, home life, finances and service wearing you down? If you answered yes to any of these questions, chances are worry is adding to your stress level and taking a toll on your health, happiness and effectiveness. But it doesn't have to be that way—God has a plan for you.

Cast all your anxiety on him because he cares for you. 1 Peter 5:7

God's Word repeatedly tells us not to worry or be anxious. Read the following verses, substituting your name in the blanks:

_____, do not be anxious about anything, but in everything, by prayer and petition, with thanksgiving, present your requests to God. And the peace of God, which transcends all understanding, will guard your heart and mind in Christ Jesus (see Philippians 4:6-7).

_____, peace I leave with you; my peace I give you. I do not give to you as the world gives. _____, do not let your heart be troubled and do not be afraid (see John 14:27).

Meditate on these verses. Breathe deeply as you think about "peace," "do not be anxious" and "do not let your [heart] be troubled." Try to fill your lungs from the top to the bottom, and as you breathe out, feel your muscles relax. Chances are you're feeling better already: physically, mentally, emotionally and spiritually. What you're experiencing is the relaxation response—God's design for helping the body overcome the effects of worry, stress and anxiety.

Count the Cost

The stress and strain of worry

- Draw your focus away from God
- Interfere with your relationships
- Affect you mentally, emotionally, spiritually and physically
- Leave you feeling fatigued
- Suppress the immune system
- Cause headaches, digestive problems, sleeplessness and depression
- Might also encourage unhealthy habits such as poor nutrition and physical inactivity

Identify the Worries in Your Life

Many things in life cause worry, stress and anxiety. Many times our worries are very real: pressures at work, too much responsibility at home and financial difficulties. Other times worry only exists in the mind and imagination. However, too often we worry about things that will never come to pass.

What things cause you to feel stressed or worried? Are you doing all you can to eliminate or respond positively to the worries in your life? Are you trusting God to deliver you from your worries? God never promises that you will not experience difficult times, but He does offer a way out.

Come to me, all you who are weary and burdened, and I will give you rest. Take my yoke upon you and learn from me, for I am gentle and humble in heart, and you will find rest for your souls. For my yoke is easy and my burden is light. Matthew 11:28-30

A Plan for Winning over Worry

God's prescription for overcoming worry is found in His Word—the Bible. Here are some things you can do to take control of the worry and stress in your life.

Take Life One Day at a Time

Therefore do not worry about tomorrow, for tomorrow will worry about itself. Each day has enough trouble of its own. Matthew 6:34

Are you managing your time well? Are your goals in line with God's purpose for your life? Are you making time in your life for the important things? In Matthew 6:34 Jesus doesn't tell us not to *think* about tomorrow; He tells us not to *worry* about tomorrow! Planning and preparing will help eliminate stress and worry. Keeping a calendar or schedule can help you control stress and organize your time. Learn to say no more often and eliminate those things that are less important. Keep the big picture of your life in front of you and don't get discouraged by the small setbacks that happen along the way.

Take Time to Rest and Relax

Come with me by yourselves to a quiet place and get some rest. Mark 6:31

Are you taking time each day for rest and relaxation? Take at least 15 to 20 minutes every day to do something relaxing: sit quietly, breathe deeply, take a walk, read, meditate and/or pray. The relaxation exercise at the beginning of this article is a great way to get started. Choose meaningful Scripture verses that work for you. Progressive relaxation involves tightening and relaxing each muscle group in your body as you lie comfortably and breathe deeply. You can also use mental imagery to relax—imagine a soothing scene in your mind while listening to peaceful music. Choose what works best for you.

Take Care of Yourself

Do you not know that your body is a temple of the Holy Spirit, who is in you, whom you have received from God? You are not your own; you were bought at a price. Therefore honor God with your body. 1 Corinthians 6:19-20

Are you making time for regular physical activity, following a healthy eating plan and getting adequate sleep? Do your poor health habits or feelings about your body contribute to the worry in your life? Physical activity is a great way to relieve stress and worry. A physically fit body responds better to the stresses of life. Regular endurance exercise may even trigger the relaxation response by releasing feel-good hormones called endorphins. Do what you enjoy: walk, swim, ride a bike or jog. Any activity that gets your muscles moving and increases your heart rate can be helpful.

Build Supportive Relationships

A friend loves at all times, and a brother is born for adversity. Proverbs 17:17

Do you have a close network of family and friends who can help you in time of stress? Sharing your worries can make you feel better and help you put things in perspective. Make sure you establish supportive relationships with *positive* people to help you in times of stress. Share your burdens and concerns with others and ask for help when you need it.

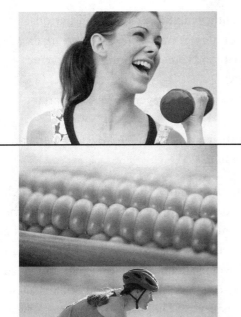

spiritual

WELL-
BEING

the faith factor

Recent polls indicate that most Americans believe in the healing power of faith and prayer.

- Nearly 80 percent believe that faith, religious practice and personal prayer can speed or help the medical treatment of people who are ill.
- More than 77 percent believe that God sometimes intervenes to cure people who have a serious illness.
- Over 60 percent say that religion and daily prayer are very important in their life.
- Sixty percent say they pray for their own health, and over 80 percent say they pray for the health of others.[1]

Faith and prayer are good for the body, mind and soul. Recent research suggests that faith is an important factor in the prevention of disease and the promotion of health. According to recent scientific evidence, over 78 scientific studies show that religious commitment is beneficial to health and well-being.[2]

A 1997 study of 5,000 men and women found that those who attended religious services frequently were 25 percent less likely to die over 28 years of follow-up as those who attended less frequently. They were also more likely to quit smoking, increase exercise, increase social contacts and have better marriages.[3]

One study found that people who attend church regularly have 50 percent less risk of dying from heart disease and 56 percent less risk of dying from lung disease compared to those who rarely go to church. They also had 74 percent less risk of dying from liver disease and 53 percent less risk of dying from suicide.[4]

Several studies show that faith has beneficial effects on blood pressure. A study of over 4,000 people aged 65 and older found that those who attended religious services at least once a week and prayed or studied the Bible at least daily had consistently lower blood pressure than those who did so less frequently or not at all.[5]

One study found that older patients who attended religious services once a week or more cut their risk of being hospitalized in the previous year by 56 percent compared to patients who attended less frequently. Hospitalized patients with a religious affiliation cut their hospital stay in half compared to those without an affiliation.[6]

The following questions are similar to the types of questions asked in the research studies previously mentioned:

• How often do you attend church or other worship services?

☐ More than once a week   ☐ Once a week
☐ A few times a month   ☐ A few times a year
☐ Once a year or less   ☐ Never

• How often do you spend time in personal religious activities, such as prayer, meditation and Bible study?

☐ More than once a day   ☐ Daily
☐ Two or more times a week   ☐ Once a week
☐ A few times a month   ☐ Rarely or never

• My Christian faith is what lies behind my whole approach to life.

☐ Definitely true of me   ☐ Tends to be true
☐ Unsure   ☐ Tends not to be true
☐ Definitely not true

• I try hard to carry my Christian faith over into all other dealings in my life.

☐ Definitely true of me   ☐ Tends to be true
☐ Unsure   ☐ Tends not to be true
☐ Definitely not true

• My Christian faith is an important source of strength and comfort in my life.

☐ Definitely true of me   ☐ Tends to be true
☐ Unsure   ☐ Tends not to be true
☐ Definitely not true

There are three additional questions you must also ask.

1. *Do I understand that good health requires balance in all areas of my life?*
2. *Am I willing to open myself up to the spiritual support of others?*
3. *How does my faith influence my daily habits and choices?*

A strong faith and regular prayer do not guarantee you will live a long life or be free from disease; they simply lower your risk. It's important to know that emotional stress and physical illness are not forms of divine punishment. God loves you and desires the very best for you (see Romans 8:31-32). However, your daily choices can have a strong influence on your overall health and well-being. Your personal faith can be a strong motivator for healthy and purposeful living.

For further information on the influence of faith on your physical health, check out the National Institutes for Healthcare Research website at www.nihr.org.

Notes
1. Source unknown.
2. National Institute for Healthcare Research.
3. *American Journal of Public Health*, Vol. 87, 1997.
4. *International Journal of Psychology in Medicine*, Vol. 28, 1998.
5. Ibid.
6. Source unknown.

hiding God's word in your heart

I have hidden your word in my heart that I might not sin against you.

Psalm 119:11

The Value of Scripture Memory

Scripture memory is an important part of the Christian life. The following are three reasons to memorize Scripture:

1. **Handling Difficult Situations**—A heartfelt knowledge of God's Word equips us to handle any situation that we might face. Declaring such truth as "I can do everything through Christ" (see Philippians 4:13) and "He will never desert me nor forsake me" (see Hebrews 13:5) will enable us to walk through situations with peace and courage.

2. **Overcoming Temptation**—Luke 4:1-13 describes how Jesus used Scripture to overcome His temptation in the desert. Knowledge of Scripture and the strength that comes with the ability to use it are an important part of putting on the full armor of God in preparation for spiritual warfare (see Ephesians 6:10-18).

3. **Getting Guidance**—Psalm 119:105 states that the Word of God is a "lamp to my feet and a light for my path." Learn to hide God's Word in your heart so that His light can direct your decisions and actions throughout your day.

What to Memorize

Memorize Scriptures that are related to an area in your life that needs growth and truth for encouragement—prayer, forgiveness, salvation, strength, overcoming temptation, rest, worry, etc. Use a concordance to find verses on those topics that have particular meaning to you. File your verses based on these topics so that you can find them when you need them. As you read God's Word, jot down meaningful verses to add to your memory file. Write the verses on index cards to have them at hand when you want to learn the verses.

To help as you begin, read Proverbs 15:23; then think back to a difficult situation in the past. Can you recall a particular verse or passage of Scripture that helped pull you through or that you used to encourage someone else? Do you have the verse memorized? If not, find the verse in your Bible, write it down and plan to memorize it.

Think back to a time when God's Word provided a way out for you. Read 1 Corinthians 10:13. Can you recall the particular verse that helped you? Do you have this verse memorized? If not, find the verse in your Bible, write it down and add it to your list of verses to be memorized.

After reading Isaiah 30:21, think back to a time when a specific verse or passage of Scripture helped you discover God's will for a particular situation. Do you have this verse memorized? If not, find the verse in your Bible, write it down and commit it to memory.

How to Memorize Scripture

Anyone can memorize Scripture. However, it does take a commitment of time and a willing heart. To memorize Scripture you must have a positive attitude and say with Paul, "I can do everything through him who gives me strength" (Philippians 4:13).

- Write the verse several times and read it aloud as you write it.
- Personalize the verse by putting your name in key places and say it in your own words. This will give you ownership of the verse and will help you apply it to your life.
- Seek to understand the verse by reading it in context. Study the verse and those surrounding it to understand what it means.
- To learn the reference (where the verse is found in the Bible), *glue* it to the first few words of the verse. When you say the verse, always say the reference before and after each recitation.
- Memorize the verse one phrase at a time. Dividing up the verse into its most meaningful components helps make the memorization process easier. Continue until you are able to quote the entire verse, word for word.
- Memorize Scripture with a family member or friend. Partnering with someone provides a fun component and a source of accountability.
- Try to review your verses daily for several months. Then review your verses at least once a month to keep them fresh in your mind.
- Use memory aids such as the First Place Scripture memory program which includes the *Walking in the Word* easel book and the Scripture

Memory music CDs or cassettes. Keep the book with you to review throughout the day. Listen to the CD or cassette as you exercise or drive.

- Make your own memory verse book by using a spiral-bound book of index cards on which you have written your own selection of verses. Practice the verses while exercising or driving. Put the written verses in convenient places and recite them whenever you get the chance.

Through a lifestyle of memorizing Scripture, the Holy Spirit will be able to bring the truth to your mind in difficult times, when temptation comes or when seeking guidance for your life. God's Spirit will also bring you opportunities to share Scripture with others whether as a witness to them or to encourage them. Remember, as you hide God's Word in your heart, you will truly be storing up treasures in heaven!

How to Make the Most of Bible Study

- Set aside time each day to spend in Bible study. There are many studies available at Christian bookstores, but you can also study God's Word on your own.
- Pray before each day's study. Ask God to give you understanding and a teachable heart.
- Stay focused. Keep in mind that the ultimate goal of Bible study is not for knowledge only but also for application and a changed life.
- If at all possible, develop accountability relationships with other believers. A weekly Bible study is an ideal way to be accountable, but if you are unable to attend a weekly meeting, find at least one other believer to keep yourself accountable.

making time for bible study and prayer

In the middle of our busy lives, we often forget that our relationship with God is the foundation from which we grow. The Great Commandment (see Mark 12:28-31) calls us into relationship with Him. Christ is the One for whom you were created (see Colossians 1:15-20), and it is He who gives you strength (see Philippians 4:13). Like any other relationship, however, it takes time and commitment to develop. The time you spend in prayer and in the Word will help you develop intimacy with God and deepen your relationship with Him.

Daily devotions and prayer are lifelines in a hectic world, especially when trying to make lifestyle changes. In the middle of the whirlwind, we can hear Jesus say, "Come away to a quiet place my child, and rest for awhile." He spoke similar words to His disciples (see Matthew 11:28); He beckons you to do the same. Your Savior calls you to steal away and spend time with Him. Will you accept His invitation?

Tailoring Your Time

Having a quiet time is a discipline that must be developed through practice and work. Deep relationships are always intentional. They require time and effort. There are no rules regarding when to do your quiet time; choose what works best for you. Find times and places that will allow you to give the Lord your undivided attention. Perhaps it is in the morning before everyone gets up. It may be in the evening after the children are in bed. Maybe noon is a time when you can get away to be with the Lord.

You also need to learn how you best communicate with Him. Remember that every relationship is unique. Tailor your quiet times to reflect your personal relationship with God.

- **What is your best time of the day for quiet time and prayer?** For some that might be early morning before others are awake, for others in the evening or even at lunchtime.
- **How much time do you have to spend on devotions?** Once you've decided on the best time, write it down on your calendar or in your daily planner in order to establish a routine. Just as with exercise and

other lifestyle changes, many people try to do too much too soon. Set aside an amount of time that works for you. Adjust your schedule as you learn what works best.

Communing with God

Take some time to learn how you best communicate and listen to God. It may even be different on different days or at different times of the day. Learn what works best for you.

- **How do you best communicate with God?** Whether through writing, talking, singing or playing music, meditating or other methods, try a variety of ways to spend time with Him.
- **Where is your favorite place to meet with God?** When you spend time with God, you need to be able to relax and focus your attention. It's important to find a special place where you're comfortable. In Matthew 6:6, Jesus said: "When you pray, go into your room, close the door and pray to your Father, who is unseen. Then your Father, who sees what is done in secret, will reward you."

Studying God's Word

There are lots of great ways to study and meditate on God's Word. For variety consider the following:

- Use a daily devotional as your guide.
- Follow a systematic plan for reading through the Bible.
- Use a Bible with study notes or other references.
- Meditate on and study a favorite verse, passage of Scripture or hymn.
- Get involved in a study group or with an accountability partner and study together, and establish a reading or devotion schedule.
- If you have a long commute to work, listening to the Bible on cassette is an excellent way to spend quality time with the Lord.
- You will probably develop other creative ideas as you continue to study.

Be prepared before you begin by gathering materials ahead of time and keep them in a specific place. Or if you like to move around, keep your Bible study materials in a basket, box or other container so that you can keep everything together. In addition to keeping a Bible, notebook and pen or pencil nearby, consider adding a Bible dictionary, other Bible translations, a hymnal or song-book, a journal, a devotional book and anything else you might find helpful. These resources can add variety to your quiet time and having them easily available will encourage you to spend more time studying and praying.

Using a Prayer List

Keeping and organizing a prayer list can help you focus your prayers on those issues that are most important. When your mind wanders, use your list to get you back on track. Write down the important issues and concerns in your life. Keep an ongoing list of people who need prayer. Other areas for prayer might include world issues, governmental leaders, missionaries and ministries. Writing down when those prayers were answered is a great encouragement to continue to pray.

Keeping a Journal

Keeping a spiritual journal is a concrete way to keep in touch with God and what's going on in your life. Keep a record of prayer requests, answered prayers and other ways God is working in your life and the lives of those around you. As time goes on, you will have a memorial of your journey with Him. Journals help to personalize your devotional time and keep you motivated.

Overcoming Roadblocks

Like any discipline, there are obstacles and roadblocks to making quiet time and prayer a part of your daily routine. Do any of these excuses sound familiar?

- I don't know where to begin.
- I don't know how or what to pray.
- I don't have time.
- I can't seem to keep myself motivated.
- The Bible is confusing to me sometimes.

What are your barriers to quiet time and prayer? How can you overcome them? Talk about your needs and brainstorm solutions with family, friends or a Bible study group. Do not forget that quiet time is a discipline to be developed; give yourself time to learn and grow. Even when you don't feel like it, make it a priority to get into the Word and spend some time with your heavenly Father. You'll be glad you did.

scripture reading plan

The following plan will guide you through an Old Testament and New Testament passage each day. You will read through the Bible in one year if you follow this plan. Each reading will take approximately 15-30 minutes to complete.

January

1 Genesis 1—3; Matthew 1
2 Genesis 4—6; Matthew 2:1-12
3 Genesis 7—8; Matthew 2:13-23
4 Genesis 9—11; Matthew 3
5 Genesis 12—14; Matthew 4:1-11
6 Genesis 15—17; Matthew 4:12-25
7 Genesis 18—19; Matthew 5:1-16
8 Genesis 20—22; Matthew 5:17-48
9 Genesis 23—24; Matthew 6:1-18
10 Genesis 25—27; Matthew 6:19-34
11 Genesis 28—29; Matthew 7:1-14
12 Genesis 30—31; Matthew 7:15-29
13 Genesis 32—33; Matthew 8:1-17
14 Genesis 34—36; Matthew 8:18-34
15 Genesis 37—38; Matthew 9:1-26
16 Genesis 39—40; Matthew 9:27-38
17 Genesis 41—42; Matthew 10
18 Genesis 43—45; Matthew 11:1-19
19 Genesis 46—47; Matthew 11:20-30
20 Genesis 48—50; Matthew 12:1-21
21 Exodus 1—2; Matthew 12:22-50
22 Exodus 3—4; Matthew 13:1-23
23 Exodus 5—7; Matthew 13:24-58
24 Exodus 8—9; Matthew 14:1-21
25 Exodus 10—11; Matthew 14:22-36
26 Exodus 12—13; Matthew 15:1-20
27 Exodus 14—15; Matthew 15:21-39
28 Exodus 16—18; Matthew 16:1-12
29 Exodus 19—21; Matthew 16:13-28
30 Exodus 22—23; Matthew 17:1-13
31 Exodus 24—26; Matthew 17:14-27

February

1 Exodus 27—28; Matthew 18:1-20
2 Exodus 29—30; Matthew 18:21-35
3 Exodus 31—32; Matthew 19:1-15
4 Exodus 33—34; Matthew 19:16-30
5 Exodus 35—36; Matthew 20:1-16
6 Exodus 37—38; Matthew 20:17-34
7 Exodus 39—40; Matthew 21:1-22
8 Leviticus 1—3; Matthew 21:23-46
9 Leviticus 4—5; Matthew 22:1-14
10 Leviticus 6—8; Matthew 22:15-46
11 Leviticus 9—10; Matthew 23
12 Leviticus 11—13; Matthew 24:1-31
13 Leviticus 14—15; Matthew 24:32-51
14 Leviticus 16—18; Matthew 25:1-30
15 Leviticus 19—20; Matthew 25:31-46
16 Leviticus 21—23; Matthew 26:1-35
17 Leviticus 24—25; Matthew 26:36-56
18 Leviticus 26—27; Matthew 26:57-75
19 Numbers 1—2; Matthew 27:1-31
20 Numbers 3—4; Matthew 27:32-66
21 Numbers 5—6; Matthew 28
22 Numbers 7; Mark 1:1-15
23 Numbers 8—10; Mark 1:16-45
24 Numbers 11—12; Mark 2:1-12
25 Numbers 13—14; Mark 2:13-28
26 Numbers 15—16; Mark 3:1-12
27 Numbers 17—18; Mark 3:13-35
28 Numbers 19—20; Mark 4:1-20
29 Numbers 21; Mark 4:21-41

March

1   Numbers 22—24; Mark 5:1-20
2   Numbers 25—26; Mark 5:21-43
3   Numbers 27—29; Mark 6:1-13
4   Numbers 30—31; Mark 6:14-32
5   Numbers 32—33; Mark 6:33-56
6   Numbers 34—36; Mark 7:1-23
7   Deuteronomy 1—2; Mark 7:24-37
8   Deuteronomy 3—4; Mark 8:1-10
9   Deuteronomy 5—6; Mark 8:11-26
10 Deuteronomy 7—9; Mark 8:27-38
11 Deuteronomy 10—11; Mark 9:1-13
12 Deuteronomy 12—14; Mark 9:14-29
13 Deuteronomy 15—17; Mark 9:30-50
14 Deuteronomy 18—20; Mark 10:1-16
15 Deuteronomy 21—23; Mark 10:17-31
16 Deuteronomy 24—26; Mark 10:32-52
17 Deuteronomy 27—28; Mark 11:1-11
18 Deuteronomy 29—30; Mark 11:12-33
19 Deuteronomy 31—32; Mark 12:1-12
20 Deuteronomy 33—34; Mark 12:13-27
21 Joshua 1—2; Mark 12:28-44
22 Joshua 3—4; Mark 13:1-13
23 Joshua 5—6; Mark 13:14-37
24 Joshua 7—8; Mark 14:1-11
25 Joshua 9—10; Mark 14:12-31
26 Joshua 11—12; Mark 14:32-52
27 Joshua 13—15; Mark 14:53-72
28 Joshua 16—18; Mark 15:1-15
29 Joshua 19—20; Mark 15:16-39
30 Joshua 21—22; Mark 15:40-47
31 Joshua 23—24; Mark 16

April

1   Judges 1—3; Luke 1:1-25
2   Judges 4—5; Luke 1:26-38
3   Judges 6; Luke 1:39-56
4   Judges 7—8; Luke 1:57-80
5   Judges 9; Luke 2:1-20
6   Judges 10—12; Luke 2:21-40
7   Judges 13—15; Luke 2:41-52
8   Judges 16; Luke 3:1-20
9   Judges 17—18; Luke 3:21-38
10 Judges 19—20; Luke 4:1-13
11 Judges 21; Luke 4:14-32
12 Ruth 1—2; Luke 4:33-44
13 Ruth 3—4; Luke 5:1-26
14 1 Samuel 1—2; Luke 5:27-39
15 1 Samuel 3—4; Luke 6:1-11
16 1 Samuel 5—6; Luke 6:12-49
17 1 Samuel 7—8; Luke 7:1-17
18 1 Samuel 9—10; Luke 7:18-35
19 1 Samuel 11—13; Luke 7:36-50
20 1 Samuel 14—15; Luke 8:1-18
21 1 Samuel 16—17; Luke 8:19-39
22 1 Samuel 18—19; Luke 8:40-56
23 1 Samuel 20—21; Luke 9:1-17
24 1 Samuel 22—23; Luke 9:18-45
25 1 Samuel 24—25; Luke 9:46-62
26 1 Samuel 26—27; Luke 10:1-24
27 1 Samuel 28—29; Luke 10:25-42
28 1 Samuel 30—31; Luke 11:1-13
29 2 Samuel 1—2; Luke 11:14-28
30 2 Samuel 3—4; Luke 11:29-54

May

1	2 Samuel 5—6; Luke 12:1-12
2	2 Samuel 7—8; Luke 12:13-34
3	2 Samuel 9—10; Luke 12:35-59
4	2 Samuel 11—12; Luke 13:1-17
5	2 Samuel 13—14; Luke 13:18-35
6	2 Samuel 15—16; Luke 14:1-24
7	2 Samuel 17—18; Luke 14:25-35
8	2 Samuel 19—20; Luke 15
9	2 Samuel 21—22; Luke 16:1-18
10	2 Samuel 23—24; Luke 16:19-31
11	1 Kings 1—2; Luke 17:1-19
12	1 Kings 3—4; Luke 17:20-37
13	1 Kings 5—6; Luke 18:1-17
14	1 Kings 7—8; Luke 18:18-43
15	1 Kings 9—11; Luke 19:1-27
16	1 Kings 12—13; Luke 19:28-48
17	1 Kings 14—15; Luke 20:1-26
18	1 Kings 16—17; Luke 20:27-47
19	1 Kings 18—19; Luke 21:1-28
20	1 Kings 20—21; Luke 21:29-38
21	1 Kings 22; Luke 22:1-23
22	2 Kings 1—3; Luke 22:24-53
23	2 Kings 4—5; Luke 22:54-71
24	2 Kings 6—7; Luke 23:1-12
25	2 Kings 8—9; Luke 23:13-32
26	2 Kings 10—11; Luke 23:33-56
27	2 Kings 12—13; Luke 24:1-12
28	2 Kings 14—15; Luke 24:13-53
29	2 Kings 16—17; John 1:1-18
30	2 Kings 18—20; John 1:19-51
31	2 Kings 21—23; John 2

June

1	2 Kings 24—25; John 3:1-21
2	1 Chronicles 1—2; John 3:22-36
3	1 Chronicles 3—4; John 4:1-42
4	1 Chronicles 5—6; John 4:43-54
5	1 Chronicles 7—8; John 5:1-17
6	1 Chronicles 9—10; John 5:18-47
7	1 Chronicles 11—12; John 6:1-15
8	1 Chronicles 13—15; John 6:16-40
9	1 Chronicles 16—17; John 6:41-71
10	1 Chronicles 18—19; John 7:1-36
11	1 Chronicles 20—21; John 7:37-52
12	1 Chronicles 22—24; John 8:1-11
13	1 Chronicles 25—27; John 8:12-59
14	1 Chronicles 28—29; John 9
15	2 Chronicles 1—2; John 10:1-21
16	2 Chronicles 3—4; John 10:22-42
17	2 Chronicles 5—6; John 11
18	2 Chronicles 7—9; John 12:1-19
19	2 Chronicles 10—12; John 12:20-50
20	2 Chronicles 13—16; John 13
21	2 Chronicles 17—19; John 14
22	2 Chronicles 20—21; John 15
23	2 Chronicles 22—23; John 16
24	2 Chronicles 24—25; John 17
25	2 Chronicles 26—27; John 18
26	2 Chronicles 28—29; John 19:1-16
27	2 Chronicles 30—31; John 19:17-42
28	2 Chronicles 32; John 20:1-18
29	2 Chronicles 33—34; John 20:19-31
30	2 Chronicles 35—36; John 21

July

1	Ezra 1—2; Acts 1
2	Ezra 3—4; Acts 2
3	Ezra 5—6; Acts 3
4	Ezra 7—8; Acts 4:1-22
5	Ezra 9—10; Acts 4:23-37
6	Nehemiah 1—3; Acts 5
7	Nehemiah 4—6; Acts 6
8	Nehemiah 7—9; Acts 7
9	Nehemiah 10—11; Acts 8:1-25
10	Nehemiah 12—13; Acts 8:26-40
11	Esther 1—2; Acts 9:1-22
12	Esther 3—6; Acts 9:23-43
13	Esther 7—10; Acts 10:1-23
14	Job 1—3; Acts 10:24-48
15	Job 4—7; Acts 11
16	Job 8—10; Acts 12
17	Job 11—14; Acts 13:1-13
18	Job 15—17; Acts 13:14-52
19	Job 18—21; Acts 14
20	Job 22—24; Acts 15
21	Job 25—28; Acts 16:1-15
22	Job 29—31; Acts 16:16-40
23	Job 32—34; Acts 17:1-15
24	Job 35—37; Acts 17:16-34
25	Job 38—39; Acts 18
26	Job 40—42; Acts 19:1-20
27	Psalms 1—6; Acts 19:21-41
28	Psalms 7—12; Acts 20:1-16
29	Psalms 13—18; Acts 20:17-38
30	Psalms 19—24; Acts 21:1-16
31	Psalms 25—30; Acts 21:17-40

August

1	Psalms 31—36; Acts 22
2	Psalms 37—41; Acts 23
3	Psalms 42—47; Acts 24
4	Psalms 48—53; Acts 25
5	Psalms 54—58; Acts 26
6	Psalms 59—64; Acts 27
7	Psalms 65—68; Acts 28:1-15
8	Psalms 69—72; Acts 28:16-31
9	Psalms 73—77; Romans 1:1-17
10	Psalms 78—80; Romans 1:18-32
11	Psalms 81—86; Romans 2
12	Psalms 87—89; Romans 3
13	Psalms 90—95; Romans 4
14	Psalms 96—102; Romans 5
15	Psalms 103—106; Romans 6
16	Psalms 107—111; Romans 7
17	Psalms 112—118; Romans 8:1-17
18	Psalms 119:1—88; Romans 8:18-39
19	Psalms 119:89—176; Romans 9
20	Psalms 120—129; Romans 10
21	Psalms 130—136; Romans 11
22	Psalms 137—140; Romans 12
23	Psalms 141—145; Romans 13
24	Psalms 146—150; Romans 14
25	Proverbs 1—3; Romans 15
26	Proverbs 4—6; Romans 16
27	Proverbs 7—9; 1 Corinthians 1
28	Proverbs 10—12; 1 Corinthians 2
29	Proverbs 13—14; 1 Corinthians 3
30	Proverbs 15—17; 1 Corinthians 4
31	Proverbs 18—20; 1 Corinthians 5

September

1 Proverbs 21—23; 1 Corinthians 6
2 Proverbs 24—26; 1 Corinthians 7
3 Proverbs 27—29; 1 Corinthians 8
4 Proverbs 30—31; 1 Corinthians 9
5 Ecclesiastes 1—3; 1 Corinthians 10
6 Ecclesiastes 4—7; 1 Corinthians 11
7 Ecclesiastes 8—12; 1 Corinthians 12
8 Song of Songs 1—4; 1 Corinthians 13
9 Song of Songs 5—8; 1 Corinthians 14
10 Isaiah 1—4; 1 Corinthians 15
11 Isaiah 5—7; 1 Corinthians 16
12 Isaiah 8—9; 2 Corinthians 1
13 Isaiah 10—12; 2 Corinthians 2
14 Isaiah 13—14; 2 Corinthians 3
15 Isaiah 15—18; 2 Corinthians 4
16 Isaiah 19—22; 2 Corinthians 5
17 Isaiah 23—25; 2 Corinthians 6
18 Isaiah 26—29; 2 Corinthians 7
19 Isaiah 30—32; 2 Corinthians 8
20 Isaiah 33—35; 2 Corinthians 9
21 Isaiah 36—39; 2 Corinthians 10
22 Isaiah 40—41; 2 Corinthians 11
23 Isaiah 42—43; 2 Corinthians 12
24 Isaiah 44—47; 2 Corinthians 13
25 Isaiah 48—50; Galatians 1
26 Isaiah 51—53; Galatians 2
27 Isaiah 54—57; Galatians 3
28 Isaiah 58—60; Galatians 4
29 Isaiah 61—63; Galatians 5
30 Isaiah 64—66; Galatians 6

October

1 Jeremiah 1; Ephesians 1
2 Jeremiah 2; Ephesians 2
3 Jeremiah 3—4; Ephesians 3
4 Jeremiah 5—6; Ephesians 4
5 Jeremiah 7—8; Ephesians 5
6 Jeremiah 9—10; Ephesians 6
7 Jeremiah 11—12; Philippians 1
8 Jeremiah 13—14; Philippians 2
9 Jeremiah 15—17; Philippians 3
10 Jeremiah 18—19; Philippians 4
11 Jeremiah 20—21; Colossians 1
12 Jeremiah 22—23; Colossians 2
13 Jeremiah 24—25; Colossians 3
14 Jeremiah 26; Colossians 4
15 Jeremiah 27—28; 1 Thessalonians 1
16 Jeremiah 29—30; 1 Thessalonians 2
17 Jeremiah 31; 1 Thessalonians 3
18 Jeremiah 32; 1 Thessalonians 4
19 Jeremiah 33—34; 1 Thessalonians 5
20 Jeremiah 35—36; 2 Thessalonians 1
21 Jeremiah 37—38; 2 Thessalonians 2
22 Jeremiah 39—41; 2 Thessalonians 3
23 Jeremiah 42—43; 1 Timothy 1
24 Jeremiah 44—45; 1 Timothy 2
25 Jeremiah 46—47; 1 Timothy 3
26 Jeremiah 48; 1 Timothy 4
27 Jeremiah 49; 1 Timothy 5
28 Jeremiah 50; 1 Timothy 6
29 Jeremiah 51; 2 Timothy 1
30 Jeremiah 52; 2 Timothy 2
31 Lamentations 1; 2 Timothy 3

November

1	Lamentations 2; 2 Timothy 4
2	Lamentations 3; Titus 1
3	Lamentations 4; Titus 2
4	Lamentations 5; Titus 3
5	Ezekiel 1—2; Philemon
6	Ezekiel 3—5; Hebrews 1
7	Ezekiel 6—7; Hebrews 2
8	Ezekiel 8—10; Hebrews 3
9	Ezekiel 11—12; Hebrews 4
10	Ezekiel 13—14; Hebrews 5
11	Ezekiel 15—16; Hebrews 6
12	Ezekiel 17—18; Hebrews 7
13	Ezekiel 19—20; Hebrews 8
14	Ezekiel 21—22; Hebrews 9
15	Ezekiel 23—24; Hebrews 10
16	Ezekiel 25—26; Hebrews 11
17	Ezekiel 27—28; Hebrews 12
18	Ezekiel 29—30; Hebrews 13
19	Ezekiel 31—32; James 1
20	Ezekiel 33—34; James 2
21	Ezekiel 35—37; James 3
22	Ezekiel 38—39; James 4
23	Ezekiel 40—41; James 5
24	Ezekiel 42—43; 1 Peter 1
25	Ezekiel 44—46; 1 Peter 2
26	Ezekiel 47—48; 1 Peter 3
27	Daniel 1; 1 Peter 4
28	Daniel 2; 1 Peter 5
29	Daniel 3; 2 Peter 1
30	Daniel 4; 2 Peter 2

December

1	Daniel 5—6; 2 Peter 3
2	Daniel 7—8; 1 John 1
3	Daniel 9; 1 John 2
4	Daniel 10—12; 1 John 3
5	Hosea 1—3; 1 John 4
6	Hosea 4—6; 1 John 5
7	Hosea 7—8; 2 John
8	Hosea 9—10; 3 John
9	Hosea 11—12; Jude
10	Hosea 13—14; Revelation 1
11	Joel; Revelation 2
12	Amos 1—2; Revelation 3
13	Amos 3—4; Revelation 4
14	Amos 5—7; Revelation 5
15	Amos 8—9; Revelation 6
16	Obadiah; Revelation 7
17	Jonah; Revelation 8
18	Micah 1—2; Revelation 9
19	Micah 3—4; Revelation 10
20	Micah 5—7; Revelation 11
21	Nahum; Revelation 12
22	Habakkuk; Revelation 13
23	Zephaniah; Revelation 14
24	Haggai; Revelation 15
25	Zechariah 1—3; Revelation 16
26	Zechariah 4—5; Revelation 17
27	Zechariah 6—8; Revelation 18
28	Zechariah 9—11; Revelation 19
29	Zechariah 12—14; Revelation 20
30	Malachi 1—2; Revelation 21
31	Malachi 3—4; Revelation 22

sharing your faith

Many of the Samaritans from that town believed in [Jesus]
because of the woman's testimony.

John 4:39

Nothing is more effective in drawing someone to Jesus than sharing personal life experiences. People are more open to the good news of Jesus Christ when they see faith in action. Personal faith stories are simple and effective ways to share what Christ is doing in your life because they show firsthand how Christ makes a difference.

What is God doing in your life? When you see God at work in your life, that is your personal faith story! If you do not have a personal faith story, perhaps it is because you don't know Jesus Christ as your personal Lord and Savior. Read through "Steps to Becoming a Christian" (pp. 40-41) and begin today to give Christ first place in your life.

Creativity and preparation in using opportunities to share a word or story about Jesus are important parts of the Christian life. Is Jesus helping you in a special way? Are you achieving a level of success or peace that you haven't experienced in other attempts to lose weight, exercise regularly or eat healthier? As people see you making changes and achieving success, they may ask you how you are doing it. How will—or do—you respond?

Remember, your story is unique and it may allow others to see what Christ is doing in your life. It may help to bring Christ into the life of another person.

Personal Statements of Faith

Look for ways to express what God is doing in your life or the lives of others. Be ready to use your own personal statement of faith whenever the opportunity presents itself.

Personal statements of faith should be short and fit naturally into a conversation. They don't require or expect any action or response from the listener. The goal is not to get another person to change but simply to help you communicate who you are and what's important to you.

Here are some examples of short statements of faith that you might use when someone asks what you are doing to lose weight.

- It's amazing how Bible study and prayer are helping me lose weight and eat healthier.
- I've had a lot of support from a group I meet with at church.
- I'm relying more on God to help me make changes in my lifestyle.

Begin keeping a list of your meaningful experiences as you spend time studying God's Word and talking to Him in prayer. Also, notice what is happening in the lives of others. Use the following questions to help you prepare short personal statements and stories of faith:

- What is God doing in your life physically, emotionally and spiritually?
- How has your relationship with God changed? Is it more intimate or personal?
- How is prayer, Bible study and/or the support of others helping you achieve your goals for a healthy lifestyle?

steps to becoming a christian

The Bible Says
- We were made for God.
- God seeks a relationship with each of us.
- God yearns for us to spend eternity with Him in heaven.

The Bad News
Sin separates us from God and eliminates our hope for heaven. Sin is defined as missing what God wants for our lives. Think of a bull's-eye and arrows that have missed the center mark; sin means missing God's mark for us.

The Good News
- Jesus, God's only Son, came to Earth as a human.
- He willingly became our sacrifice by dying on the cross for our sins.
- We cannot save ourselves. Jesus' blood covers all our sins and reconciles us to God.

Have you ever made the decision to ask Jesus Christ to be your Savior?

☐ Yes ☐ No

If you answered yes, write about your personal experience. If your answer is no, you may open your heart to God now. There are four simple steps to take.

1. **Acknowledge that you are a sinner.** "For all have sinned and fall short of the glory of God" (Romans 3:23).
2. **Acknowledge that sin separates you from God.** "For the wages of sin is death, but the gift of God is eternal life in Christ Jesus our Lord" (Romans 6:23).
3. **Acknowledge that Christ died for you.** "But God demonstrates his own love for us in this: While we were still sinners, Christ died for us" (Romans 5:8).
4. **Receive Christ as Savior.** "If you confess with your mouth 'Jesus is Lord,' and believe in your heart that God raised him from the dead, you will be saved. For it is with your heart that you believe and are justified, and it is with your mouth that you confess and are saved" (Romans 10:9-10).

Now pray the following prayer, inviting Christ to become Lord over your life:

Dear God,

I know I am a sinner and separated from You. I believe You love me and that You sent Jesus to die on the cross for me. I accept Jesus as my Savior and my Lord. Please forgive me of my sin and teach me how to give You first place in my life. Amen.

Now What?

If you have prayed this prayer, you have made an important decision that you need to share with a Christian friend or pastor. The following article—"Steps for Spiritual Growth"—will help you begin the journey you have chosen to take with Jesus Christ as your Savior.

steps for spiritual growth

Prayer

- Prayer provides spiritual food and water for *daily* living.
- Prayer helps you to give your life back to God daily.
- Prayer allows you to confess your sins daily.

  If we confess our sins, he is faithful and just and will forgive us our sins and purify us from all unrighteousness. 1 John 1:9

The Bible

- Studying the Bible keeps you grounded in the essential ingredients for *daily* living.
- The Bible teaches you about the life of Jesus (read the New Testament Gospels of Matthew, Mark, Luke and John).
- The Bible assures you of your salvation.

  I write these things to you who believe in the name of the Son of God so that you may know that you have eternal life. 1 John 5:13

The Church

- The church provides fellowship with other believers and a place to worship God.
- Being baptized is the first step to obedience (Matthew 3:13-17 tells of Jesus' baptism.)
- Become a member of a Bible-teaching, Bible-believing community of believers.
- The Church is Christ's body on Earth, formed to spread the good news.

  So in Christ we who are many form one body, and each member belongs to all the others. Romans 12:5

Sharing Your Faith

• Jesus commanded us to share with others what Christ has done and how He continues to work in our lives.

> Then Jesus came to them and said, "All authority in heaven and on earth has been given to me. Therefore go and make disciples of all nations, baptizing them in the name of the Father and of the Son and of the Holy Spirit, and teaching them to obey everything I have commanded you. And surely I am with you always, to the very end of the age." Matthew 28:18-20

• Sharing your faith with others is merely telling your story—how God has changed you and how He helps you daily.

> Do not worry about how you will defend yourselves or what you will say, for the Holy Spirit will teach you at that time what you should say. Luke 12:11-12

• The Bible promises that the Holy Spirit will help you.

> But you will receive power when the Holy Spirit comes on you; and you will be my witnesses in Jerusalem, and in all Judea and Samaria, and to the ends of the earth. Acts 1:8

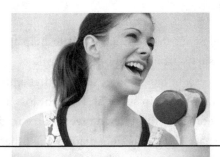

mental

WELL-
BEING

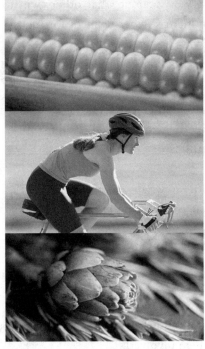

accountability partners

As iron sharpens iron, so one man sharpens another.
Proverbs 27:17

When it comes to changing our lifestyles, most of us need a little help from others. Support from family, friends, small-group members, coworkers and neighbors is important for long-term success. In fact, studies suggest that a high level of support from others is an important factor in successful weight loss and maintenance. Yet far too often, when it comes to lifestyle change, we try to do it all on our own. We're reluctant to share our goals and plans with others. Maybe it's the fear of failure. Maybe we worry about what others will think about us. Whatever the reasons, you can increase your chances for success by partnering with others to achieve your goals.

There are many reasons you may need the support of others. Here are a few of the things supportive partners can do for you.

- Provide you with advice and ideas to help you stay on track.
- Give you support and encouragement when you need them most.
- Be an important source of accountability.
- Help you keep things in perspective.
- Push you and give constructive criticism when you need it.
- Help you organize your time so that you can do the things you need to do.
- Participate and make lifestyle changes with you.

Building Your Team
The key to building your success team is finding the most supportive people you know and developing a plan to get them involved.

A Good Partner Is Someone
- With whom you feel comfortable sharing your thoughts, feelings, successes and struggles
- Who truly desires to see you succeed
- Who has a positive attitude and is a good source of encouragement and support.

- With whom you enjoy spending time
- Who will stick with you for the long-term and will always be there for you
- Who understands, values and identifies with your thoughts and feelings
- Who has been successful in making the same or similar changes that you are trying to make

How to Choose

Use the following questions when choosing a partner or evaluating the success of a partnership:

- Does your partner understand your needs, struggles and concerns?
- Are you comfortable talking openly to your partner about what's going on in your life?
- Can you communicate with your partner about specific ways that he or she can help you?
- Are you open to and willing to accept the advice, support and criticism of your partner?
- Does your partner help keep you on track by encouraging you to do things consistent with your goals?
- Is your partner committed to you for the long term and available when you need him or her?
- Does your partner avoid being critical or judgmental when you slip up or fall short of your goals?
- Is your partner happy for your successes even when he or she is not having similar success?
- Can you trust your partner to be open with you and give you honest feedback?

Who Is Not a Good Partner for Me

It's also important to know who will not make a good partner. Some partners can actually sabotage your efforts to make successful lifestyle changes. Can you think of someone who is always trying to get you to eat high-calorie foods, extra helpings or dessert? Some people may not even want to see you succeed—it makes them feel threatened. Examine your no responses to the previous questions. When choosing or thinking about a partner, the more no responses you have about that person, the less likely he or she will be a good partner for you. One or two no answers don't mean that particular person can't be your partner, but you will need to communicate your needs and concerns with this person clearly. Here are some suggestions.

- Avoid—or confront in a positive way—the people who consistently try to interfere with your efforts to lose weight and eat healthier.
- Refuse to let other people influence the decisions you make.
- Learn to say no!
- Talk openly with people to let them know how you feel and what they can do to help you. They may not know how to help.
- Kindly ask them not to tempt you with choices that don't fit in to your goals and plans.
- Be sensitive to the feelings of others; your success may make others feel insecure or threatened.
- Be a positive influence on others, rather than letting them become a negative influence on you.

Think about the people in your life—family, friends, small-group members, coworkers and neighbors. Make a list of the people who are the most influential in your efforts to lose weight and change your lifestyle. Evaluate your relationship with each of these people based on what you have learned.

building a healthy body image

When we pick up any fashion magazine, flip on the TV, and notice the billboards, what do we see? Everywhere we turn, we're presented with unrealistic images of how we should look, what we should wear and how we should live. Beautiful bodies are placed alongside ads for fattening foods, which sends the message that you *can* have it all. How do you measure up to what you see? How do these images and messages influence the way you feel about yourself? Do they influence your lifestyle habits and the goals you set for yourself? Are these messages and ideals in line with God's purpose for your life?

Don't let the media or society's unrealistic expectations influence the goals you set or the way you feel about yourself. Trying to live up to these unrealistic demands will only lead to failure, guilt and disappointment. Set your sights on the more important things in life: your relationship to God, good health and effective living.

Achieving the current ideal body image requires extremes of diet, exercise and cosmetic surgery; it's an image that often comes at the price of good health. Despite what we're led to believe, the society's version of the ideal body is outside the reach of the majority of men and women and is not a matter of self-discipline. There's absolutely no truth to the prevailing message that thinness equals health and happiness.

What the Numbers Show

- Surveys reveal that less than 15 percent of women are happy with their body weight or how they look. Women are three times more likely to be dissatisfied with their appearance than men.
- At any given time nearly 60 percent of women report being on a diet to lose weight; this includes adolescent females. Many women on diets are already at or below a normal body weight.
- Overall, nearly 65 million Americans are dieting at any one time at a cost of over $40 billion dollars each year. More than 80 percent of people who lose weight gain it all back within five years.
- A decade ago fashion models weighed 8 percent less than the average woman; today they weigh 23 percent less. The average woman is 5'4" and weighs nearly 145 pounds, while the average fashion model is 5'9" and weighs 110 pounds.
- Models and beauty-pageant contestants on average are at least 15 percent below the recommended weight for their height—one of the criteria for diagnosing an eating disorder.
- Eating disorders are on the rise—in both women and men!

Having a positive attitude and accepting who you are is the first step to making healthy lifestyle changes. It often becomes much easier to make permanent lifestyle changes once you accept the reality that you may never have a perfect body shape; the goal now becomes one of good health and better living. Take a moment to consider your reasons for wanting to lose weight.

Determining Your Success

You should primarily judge your success by how well you meet your goal for good health. Rather than focusing on the scale, set your sights on healthy eating habits and regular physical activity. If you are overweight, healthy lifestyle changes that result in a 10 percent weight loss will result in important improvements in your health and quality of life. That's enough weight loss to improve your health and quality of life but may not be enough to achieve your *ideal* body weight. The goal is not to have a perfect model's figure but to live a healthier, happier and more productive life—in the body that you have! These are achievable goals.

There's a popular quote that goes something like this: "Your body is where you'll spend the rest of your life; isn't it about time you made it your home?" Actually, isn't it about time you made it God's home (see 1 Corinthians 6:19-20) too?

healthy living on the job

Whatever you do, work at it with all your heart, as working
for the Lord, not for men, since you know that you will receive an
inheritance from the Lord as a reward.

Colossians 3:23-24

Work is a necessary part of life. It can provide both joy and satisfaction. Unfortunately, it also brings schedules, deadlines, long hours and many other responsibilities and stresses. The fast pace of work life often makes it hard to make healthful choices on the job. Pressures and responsibilities at work are common reasons people give for not taking better care of themselves.

You have to make taking care of yourself a priority while on the job. Prayerfully consider ways to make healthy living a part of your workday. Ask family, friends and coworkers to help you find creative ways to do what you need to do to stay healthy. You can generally find several minutes during the day to do something good for yourself. Look at your typical workday: Are you eating healthy? Do you make time for physical activity? How do you deal with job-related stress?

Here are some suggestions and tips to help you get started. Don't try to change everything at once. Start with those changes you're most ready to make and most confident you can change.

Eat Healthy

- Never skip meals. Your body needs food throughout the day for energy. Start your day with a nutritious breakfast and don't skip lunch. Every meal you miss robs your body of important nutrients. Also, skipping meals will make it more likely that you'll overeat later.
- Prepare and take your own food. You're much more likely to eat healthy meals and snacks if you prepare them yourself. The key is planning ahead.
  - ✓ Healthy eating at work begins at the grocery store. Make a list of foods you enjoy and that are easy for you to bring to work. Choose fresh, canned or dried fruits, raw or canned vegetables, lean sandwich meats, low-fat crackers, bean or broth-based soups, low-fat milk and yogurt.
  - ✓ Cook extra portions with evening meals and pack the leftovers for work—homemade fast food.
  - ✓ If you don't have a refrigerator at work, bring an ice cooler or insulated lunch bag. Buy plastic containers in which you can store foods and beverages.
  - ✓ Store healthy snacks in your desk drawer, briefcase or car. Low-fat crackers, graham crackers, cookies, bagels, fresh or dried fruit, cereal, popcorn and instant oatmeal are all great choices.
- When you eat out, choose your restaurants and your meals carefully.
  - ✓ Watch your portion sizes; they are usually much more than you need.
  - ✓ Split your meal with a companion or box some of it up and bring it home.
  - ✓ Avoid fried foods and dishes cooked with heavy sauces or lots of cheese. Choose bean or broth-based soups, baked or grilled chicken, fresh salads with low-fat dressing, steamed vegetables, sandwiches with lean meat and fresh fruit.
  - ✓ Find two or three restaurants where you know you can make healthy choices; recommend these when eating out.

Be More Physically Active

Fit physical activity into your workday whenever you can. Even 5 to 10 minutes of activity done throughout the day can improve your health and fitness.

- Schedule activity into your day just like you do important meetings.
- Park your car farther away from your office building.
- Take the stairs instead of the elevator.
- Use the bathroom on at least the next floor up or across the building.
- Hand deliver messages rather than use office mail, the computer or telephone.
- Take 10- to 15-minute walking breaks.
- Stand up and do some stretching while you're talking on the phone.
- Buy some handheld weights or elastic exercise bands to use in your office.
- Go for a walk during your lunch hour.
- Start a walking group or aerobic dance class at work.
- Make time for physical activity when you travel—walk in the airport between flights.
- Talk to your company about purchasing a few pieces of exercise equipment.

Reduce Stress

You may not be able to eliminate the stress of your job, but you can learn to handle it in more positive ways. Here are some tips to help you reduce and respond more positively to stress you may experience on the job. Stress often begins before you arrive at work: running late, taking care of personal responsibilities and fighting traffic.

- Get organized; do most of your preparation the night before.
- Be sure to get enough sleep. Most people need seven to nine hours of sleep every night. Discover how much sleep you need and try to get it every night.
- Arrange your schedule so that you can avoid driving in heavy traffic.
- Leave your home early enough so that you're not rushed.
- Take time to relax before you leave for work or while you're in the car: breathe deeply, relax your muscles, pray or listen to relaxing music or the Bible on cassette.
- At work, once or twice a day take 10 or 15 minutes to relax and organize the rest of your day.
- Prioritize your daily and weekly activities.

- Learn to recognize things that are less important or not important at all.
- Schedule time for yourself.
- Focus on one thing at a time.
- Learn to say "No!" or "I need help!"
- Personalize your workspace with pictures and special messages.
- Avoid cigarette smoke and limit caffeine intake.
- Friends, coworkers and family can offer encouragement and support during stressful times. Look for ways to share responsibilities with others. Think of specific things people can do to help you reduce your stress.
- Set aside time each week to discuss issues, plans, schedules and responsibilities with your family, friends and coworkers. Make this a time for teamwork and positive problem solving.
- Make sure you're making time to enjoy yourself outside of work. You need to get away and take time for yourself and loved ones.

healthy strategies for social situations

Special occasions are usually wonderful times for fellowship and enjoying good food. Unfortunately, much of the focus is on too much food and foods too high in calories, fat and sugar! Are there certain situations that cause you to give up or give in? It's not uncommon for the holidays or a special get-together to derail your healthy eating plan. Does this mean you can't have any fun at the party? Of course not! What it means is that you need to anticipate the challenges and make a plan to stick with your healthy goals. Planning ahead is the key to success!

The next time you are attending a party or special get-together, remember some basic rules for success. Before going to the party, picture in your mind how the event will go. What kinds of foods will be there? Anticipate situations and food temptations that will be difficult for you. Imagine yourself being in control of your eating and making healthy choices. Set some ground rules for yourself before you get there.

- Plan to fill your plate only one time.
- Limit yourself to small servings.
- Eat before you go, and enjoy the fellowship instead; never go to a special event hungry.
- Make up your mind to avoid the tempting high-fat, high-calorie choices.
- Ask someone to hold you accountable.
- Decide in advance that you'll only eat a few bites of your favorite food.
- Check out the available foods, and choose only one or two that are your *absolute* favorites and leave the rest behind.
- If it is a potluck event, bring a delicious low-fat version of a favorite. It just might be the hit of the party!
- Eat slowly; it takes about 20 minutes for your brain to get the message that your stomach is full.

Keep Burning the Calories

On the day (or for a day or two after) of a special occasion, make sure you fit in your physical activity. Taking a brisk walk prior to the event can help curb your appetite. Just participating in exercise helps to boost motivation and provides encouragement for managing tempting situations. Physical activity is also a great way to burn calories. You may have to exercise in the morning or at other times to guarantee you'll fit it in. Be creative and fit in physical activity however you can.

Focus on Fun and Fellowship

The relationships you build and the fun times will be much more valuable to you than any of the foods you might eat. Decide ahead of time that you'll have a meaningful conversation with several people at the gathering. Focus on others, rather than on yourself and your appetite. In fact, nutrition and health might be a good topic of conversation. Don't visit with others while standing next to the food, and try not to eat while talking with other people—hold a low-calorie beverage in your hand instead.

Success Tips for Specific Occasions

Business and Meetings

If you're in the business world, you may attend seminars, meetings and other special events. You may also have to travel. If you're not in the business world, you probably attend a lot of meetings anyway: church meetings, Bible study, community meetings and get-togethers with family and friends. Unfortunately, most of these occasions involve food. By planning ahead you can stick with your goals for a healthy lifestyle.

- Decide ahead of time to pack your own snacks: raw vegetables, fruit, low-fat crackers, pretzels or a whole-grain bagel. Bringing your own snack will provide you with a backup in case no healthy foods are offered. It's also a great way to curb your appetite if a meeting runs long.
- Make sure you drink plenty of water. Avoid high-calorie beverages, such as soft drinks and coffee with cream.
- Make time for physical activity. Sitting for hours at a time can cause boredom, which triggers snacking. Even a 5- or 10-minute walk is helpful.
- Watch out for buffet-style food service. Load up on fresh fruits, vegetables and other low-fat choices. Don't load your plate just because "it's all you can eat." Rather than trying all the foods, pick one or two of your favorites and keep your portions small.
- If you're providing the food or bringing a dish, make sure it's healthy. Don't feel you have to please people with high-fat desserts and other foods. You'll be surprised at how appreciative people will be at your thoughtfulness.

Holidays and Parties

Special occasions are celebrated with special foods! During these times, tempting foods are usually everywhere, and everyone is eating them and offering them to you. Know what situations are most difficult for you. With some simple strategies, holidays and parties can be enjoyed without the guilt of overdoing it. Here are some strategies to help get you started.

- Make a commitment to stick with your goals.
- Stick to your regular eating schedule. This will help you avoid the all-day grazing that can sometimes occur when food is always around.

- Remember to eat slowly and concentrate on enjoying the foods you eat.
- Because special foods are always around, taste small portions of the items that are truly unique to the season and leave the everyday foods alone.
- Rather than overdoing it every day, plan for one or two special meals you'll really enjoy; make up for these by eating healthy the rest of the time.
- Learn to say "No, thank you." It's okay to turn down food politely. Have a plan for what you'll say.
- Make sure you take time to relax before and during special occasions and during holidays. Spend some time praying and meditating about ways that will help you stick with your goals.
- Don't allow yourself to gain weight over the holidays; weigh yourself at least once a week. Cut back and resume your eating plan if you notice your weight creeping upward.
- Plan enjoyable activities that are not centered around food; be creative.
- If you're the host, plan to serve healthy foods. Learn to make low-fat substitutions in the recipes for some of your favorite holiday foods.
- Avoid all-or-nothing thinking; don't deprive yourself or feel guilty about enjoying certain foods.

The secret to healthy eating for special occasions is to have a plan and remember the principles of balance, moderation and variety.

managing your time

Time—there never seems to be enough of it. Yet God has given each one of us all the time we need: 60 minutes in an hour, 24 hours in a day and 168 hours in a week. Getting everything done within these time limits is quite a challenge. Obligations at home, work and church compete with less-important activities for your time. The key is focusing on the important activities and eliminating those that are not important. Some things should take priority: spending time with the Lord, taking care of yourself and serving others. Gaining control of your time helps you move through life with peace and purpose.

A Time to Change

Time—or lack of it—is one of the most common barriers Americans cite for not taking care of their bodies. What's the number-one excuse for not exercising regularly? You guessed it—lack of time! Convenience is one of the most important factors people consider when selecting a meal or including exercise in their day.

It's true that lifestyle change takes time. Unfortunately, there are no extra hours in a day. Trying to keep pace with all you have to do can be frustrating and stressful. By simplifying your life and organizing your time you can improve your health and quality of life.

Personal Time Inventory

The first step in managing your time is to know how you spend it. Use the following inventory to find out where and how you spend your time.

During the next several days evaluate how much time you actually spend in the following activities; use the extra spaces to fill in activities not on the list. Write in the hours you spend in each activity daily or weekly; choose what works best for you. Try to account for as much of the 24 hours in a day or the 168 hours in a week as possible.

Actual Time I Spend on Activities

Activity	Hrs.	Activity	Hrs.	Activity	Hrs.	Activity	Hrs.
Bible study		Grooming		Recreation		Working	
Church		Housework		Shopping			
Cooking/ dining		Paying bills		Sleeping			
Daydreaming		Physical activity		Social activities			
Driving/travel		Prayer		Telephone			
Family time		Reading		Television			

Next, use the following inventory to determine the ideal amount of time you would like to spend in each activity:

Ideal Time I Would Like to Spend on Activities

Activity	Hrs.	Activity	Hrs.	Activity	Hrs.	Activity	Hrs.
Bible study		Grooming		Recreation		Working	
Church		Housework		Shopping			
Cooking/ dining		Paying bills		Sleeping			
Daydreaming		Physical activity		Social activities			
Driving/travel		Prayer		Telephone			
Family time		Reading		Television			

Review how much time you spend in each activity. Compare this with your inventory of how much time you would ideally like to spend on each activity. See what activities are taking up too much of your time. Prayerfully ask God to help you learn where and how to make better use of your time.

Making a plan to plan is the most important step in using your time wisely. Set aside time each day to review your plans for the day and upcoming week. What is the best time of day for you? Is it in the morning? Or maybe at night? You also need to set aside several hours each month, or at least every three months, to review where you've been, what you've done and where you are going. Look at both your short- and long-term goals. What changes do you need to make? What projects have you completed and what goals have you achieved?

Time-Saving Tips

• Keep a calendar or daily organizer to keep track of all your appointments and plans. Write everything down and review it often.
• Learn to use a checklist to keep track of your day's events. Use your organizer and checklist to help you get into a routine.
• Always give yourself time to review your goals, responsibilities and schedule before adding new things. Learn to say no to things that aren't a good use of your time.
• Stick with one or two important tasks each day. Keep a wish list of things you need to do or would like to do once you finish the important tasks.

- When making your daily, weekly and long-term plans, make sure you schedule time to take care of yourself: physical activity, relaxation and fun times with family and friends.
- Don't expect everything to go perfectly; just do the best you can.
- Do the difficult things first! Try not to put off too much until tomorrow.
- Break big projects into smaller pieces. Reward yourself for completing each step.
- Learn to ask family and friends for the help you need.
- Make a list of the activities with which you need help; be specific.
- Make a list of specific people who can help you with each activity.
- Determine who can help with household chores: taking out the trash, doing dishes, mowing the grass, running errands.
- Who can help you at work? What can they do?
- Have someone hold you accountable for organizing your time. Ask them to review with you how you spend your time. Ask them to help you eliminate those activities that are less important.

A Plan to Change

What are the top three reasons you don't use your time as wisely as you would like: lack of organization, letting others control your time, too many responsibilities, wasting time, procrastination? List your reasons. Be specific!

Next, determine three steps you can take to overcome each of these time wasters. Start with the area you're most ready and confident you can change. Work through each step, trying to make each one a habit before moving on to the next.

pressing on toward the goal

But one thing I do: Forgetting what is behind and straining toward
what is ahead, I press on toward the goal to win the prize
for which God has called me heavenward in Christ Jesus.
Philippians 3:13-14

Two dictionary definitions of "goal": the ending point of a race or the end toward which effort is directed. Too often we focus on the end of the race and forget about the effort. It's easy to set goals; it's much harder to formulate a plan and accomplish the necessary steps to win the prize.

Winning Goals

Why are goals so important? Because in life we need goals to help us achieve. God clearly desires to be at the center of all our plans (see Proverbs 3:5-6; 16:9). When setting goals, the most important question we must ask ourselves is: *Is my goal in line with God's desire for my life?*

When setting lifestyle goals, consider the goal worthwhile and consistent with God's plan for your life if you can answer yes to one or more of the following questions:

- *Will achieving my goal help me grow closer to God and serve Him better?*
- *Will achieving my goal help me to feel better about myself and live more effectively?*
- *Will achieving my goal improve my ability to serve others?*
- *Will achieving my goal improve my health and well-being?*

Prayerfully seek God's wisdom and guidance before moving ahead with your goals and plans. You should also seek wise counsel from trusted family and friends. Remember, it's better to spend several weeks prayerfully considering and developing your goals and plans than it is to start tomorrow toward a goal that you can't (or shouldn't) achieve.

Setting Realistic Goals

How many times have you made up your mind that you were going to make a change and then fallen short of your goal? Do any of these sound familiar?

- I'll never eat dessert again.
- I'm going to exercise at 7 A.M. every day.
- I'm going to spend one hour daily in quiet time.
- I will lose 60 pounds in three months.

It's best to avoid setting too rigid or all-or-none goals that use words such as "never again," "always," "every day," "must," etc. Setting goals that are unrealistic or too demanding will set you up for failure and disappointment.

Another reason people often fall short of their goals is that they try to take on too much too soon. Realistic goals and a well-thought-out plan are the most important ingredients for success.

Setting Goals and Developing a Plan

The key to setting goals and building a successful plan is to ask yourself the right questions.

What Do You Want to Accomplish?

It's important to have a clear idea of where you want to go before you get started. Do you really want to achieve a certain weight or is the underlying issue that you want to feel better about yourself? When setting a goal, it's important to have a clear idea of the benefits you are looking for. Ask yourself how your life will be different when you achieve your goal. How will you feel if you don't achieve your goal?

What Are Your Motivations?

People who are successful in achieving and maintaining long-term goals have clear reasons for doing so. In other words, the reward has to be worth the effort. When setting goals, it's much more important to focus on things you can do rather than on things you wish you could be. Motivations such as improving your relationships, feeling better and improving your health are much stronger motivations than looking better or achieving an ideal body weight for a special event such as a high school reunion or wedding.

What Steps Do You Need to Take?

When setting goals it's important to have the long-term results in mind, but it's much more important to focus on what you can do each day to achieve them. It's much better to start with small goals and succeed than to start with big goals and fail because it is too overwhelming. With each success, you'll gain the confidence and encouragement you need to take the next step.

What Things Might Keep You from Reaching Your Goal?

It's important to think about situations, people and feelings that may keep you from achieving or maintaining your goals. Understanding your past successes or failures is a great place to start when setting new goals. Think about some goals you've set for yourself in the past. What worked for you and what didn't? Are you committed to achieving your goal? Are you willing to stick with your plans when times get tough or you experience a setback? It's also important to have goals and plans that are flexible. You will encounter life changes along the way; be prepared to adjust your expectations.

Who Can Help and How Can They Help You?

It's very difficult to make lifestyle changes without the support of family and friends. Having a solid system of support greatly increases your chances for success. Try to seek out people who have accomplished what you are trying to achieve. Finding family and friends who have goals similar to yours can also be helpful. This step requires some effort on your part; you will have to ask for the help you need. Don't expect people to understand your needs and volunteer their help.

How Can You Monitor Your Progress?

Self-monitoring is one of the best predictors of success when striving for a goal. The ability to see your progress along the way helps keep you motivated and on track. The path to most goals is usually not a straight line. By monitoring your progress you'll see that a slipup or two along the way can't reverse all the progress you've made. When setting goals, make sure you build in a plan for monitoring your progress. Have a plan for rewarding yourself as you achieve important victories along the way. Remember, if you don't know what you're aiming for, you'll hit it every time.

understanding weight gain and obesity

Despite an increasing emphasis on healthier lifestyles, the number of Americans who are overweight is growing rapidly. Currently 61 percent of adults are overweight or obese, and the degree of obesity in children is increasing at an alarming rate. At any one time, nearly 50 percent of men and women are trying to lose weight. Unfortunately, they are usually unsuccessful.

Is Your Weight Increasing?

Has your weight been increasing steadily over the last several years? Or have you noticed a sudden jump in your weight? What changes in your life and lifestyle may be contributing to your weight gain? One of the best things you can do for your overall health is to prevent any further weight gain. In fact, studies show that following a healthy lifestyle of good nutrition and regular physical activity is more important to your overall health and well-being than what you weigh. Committing yourself to a healthy lifestyle and maintaining your present weight are important and worthwhile goals.

Why the Increase in Being Overweight?

Most experts attribute increasing levels of obesity to the demands of modern living. Longer work hours and more time spent in the car leave less time for physical activity and healthy eating. It's not hard to see that remote controls, computers, self-propelled lawnmowers and drive-thrus have become part of everyday life. While modern technology is good, it decreases opportunities for physical activity at home and at work. Combined with easy access to a variety of high-calorie, high-fat and good-tasting foods, modern living makes it very difficult to maintain a healthy weight.

While weight gain results from an imbalance between calorie intake and energy expenditure, weight regulation is actually a complex process in which physical, hormonal, environmental, genetic, emotional and social issues can influence metabolism, appetite, body composition, activity levels and lifestyle choices.

Society's view that obesity is an issue of willpower and choice and popular diets that place the blame on certain foods or one specific cause are overly simplistic and misleading.

Considering the fact that you are most likely to be successful in changing those aspects of your lifestyle that you're ready to change and that you're most confident you can change, what changes in your environment and lifestyle are you ready to make?

The Health Risks of Being Overweight

A lifestyle of poor dietary habits and physical inactivity which results in being overweight or obese, is the second leading cause of preventable death in this country, resulting in over 300,000 deaths each year! Being overweight and obese are major risk factors for coronary heart disease and are strongly associated with several health problems, including

- Diabetes
- High cholesterol
- High blood pressure
- Cancer
- Stroke
- Arthritis
- Gallbladder disease
- Sleep problems
- Infertility

Good News!

Scientific evidence now shows that a weight loss of just 5 to 10 percent can significantly reduce—and even reverse!—the negative health effects associated with being overweight or obese. Moderate weight loss is also associated with an improved quality of life. With this new evidence, experts are abandoning the concept of "ideal" weight in favor of the term "healthier" weight.

What are your health risks? Answer the following questions honestly:

- Do you have any have any obesity-related diseases or health risks?
- If you don't know your risk factors, visit your doctor for a checkup.
- Because some diseases and risk factors don't develop until later in life, it's important to look at what problems run in your family. Do any obesity-related diseases or health risks run in your family?
- Do you believe that losing weight will help lower your risk factors?
- Are you ready to commit to losing 10 percent of your current weight (if you're overweight) to improve your health?
- Multiply your current body weight by .9 to determine your healthier weight.
- Are you willing to make the lifestyle changes necessary to achieve and maintain this weight, even if you can't achieve your ideal weight?

Losing weight and keeping it off are both difficult. Even the best weight-loss programs are associated with an average weight loss of only 10 to 15 percent—hardly enough to reach the ideal most of us would like! In fact, 60 percent of people who are initially successful in losing weight gain it back within a year; almost all gain it back within three to five years! Are your expectations realistic? Be careful not to set weight and lifestyle goals that you cannot realistically keep.

Understanding Your Healthy Weight

Many people have unrealistic expectations about their bodies and ideal body weight. We live in a society that values a lean and fit body, but a healthy weight is not necessarily the popular ideal. More important is living a healthy lifestyle and maintaining a weight that's associated with good health and abundant living. A healthy weight considers who you are emotionally, spiritually, intellectually, physically and socially. Your goal should be to follow a lifestyle that's in balance with God's overall desire for your life.

Find Your Healthy Weight

This worksheet will give you some additional tools to help you set goals and track your progress. Experts now use Body-Mass Index (BMI) to determine healthy weight. A healthy weight is not about physical appearance or a number on the scale. In most people, BMI provides an accurate reflection of body composition and health risks.

How to Calculate Your BMI
Multiply your current weight in pounds by 703
Weight _____ x 703 = (a) _____
Divide the result (a) by your height in inches
(a) _____ ÷ height _____ = (b) _____
Divide the result (b) by your height in inches
(b) _____ ÷ height _____ = BMI _____

Understanding Your BMI
< 20 —Weight loss not indicated
20 to 25 —This is your healthy weight range
26 to 30 —Increasing health risk
> 30 —Obesity and high health risk
> 40 —Very high health risk

Note: Some people who are very muscular and fit can have a high BMI yet be very lean and healthy.

Know Your Body Type—Apple or a Pear

Where you carry your weight is also related to the health risks associated with obesity. People who tend to put on weight above the waist—those who are apple shaped—have a greater chance of developing heart disease, abnormal cholesterol levels, high blood pressure and diabetes. People who carry their extra weight below the waistline—pear shaped—don't seem to have as high a risk of developing these conditions. To find out your shape and determine your risk, you can measure your waist and hips to determine your waist-to-hip ratio.

How to Determine Your Waist-to-Hip Ratio

- Measure around the smallest part of your waistline in inches; don't pull in, just stand relaxed. The narrowest part of your waistline is usually at the level of your hipbone and near your belly button.
- Next, measure your hips in inches at the widest part of your buttocks.
- Divide your waist measurement by your hip measurement:
Waist _____ ÷ hip _____ = waist-to-hip ratio _____
- A healthy waist-to-hip ratio for women is below .8 and for men below 1.0.

Know Your Waist Size

Your waist size is also a good measure of the amount of fat you carry in your abdomen. Waist size is an important indicator of health risk. A waist measurement greater than 35 inches for women and 40 inches for men indicates a much higher risk of developing weight-related health problems. Because the scale doesn't always reflect what's happening to your body weight, pay attention to your waistline. Are your clothes fitting differently? Is your waistline getting smaller? These are often better indicators of healthy weight loss than the numbers on the scale.

Avoid the Yo-Yo Effect

Healthy weight loss also involves achieving a weight and following a lifestyle that you can maintain for a lifetime. Repeated cycles of weight loss and weight gain—yo-yo dieting—are not healthy. It's important to set realistic goals. Unrealistic goals and expectations encourage unhealthy weight-loss methods, result in yo-yo dieting and set you up for failure and discouragement. It's better to achieve and maintain moderate weight loss than it is to cycle repeatedly, losing and gaining large amounts of weight. Repeated ups and downs—both on the scale and emotionally—are not the answer for good health and abundant living.

To be successful in losing weight and maintaining it for a lifetime, it's important to examine your past attempts to lose weight. Looking back at past attempts to lose weight, determine which things worked and which didn't. How ready are you to lose weight this time compared to previous attempts? Are you willing and ready to make a commitment to the permanent lifestyle changes necessary for good health and long-term weight loss?

Avoid Unrealistic or Negative Feelings About Your Body

Are you dissatisfied with your body and its shape? Do you worry a lot about your appearance? Remember that you are fearfully and wonderfully made (see Psalm 139:14). God values you! Don't let the unrealistic expectations of others influence how you think about yourself. Let God, who knows and loves you, and your own heartfelt sense of who you are determine your value and what weight is right for you.

> Be honest in your estimate of yourselves, measuring your value by how much faith
> God has given you. Romans 12:3, TLB

Unrealistic goals and expectations about weight loss and body image can lead to feelings of guilt, failure and disappointment. Prayerfully consider your thoughts and feelings about your weight. By taking your focus off the scale, you can commit yourself better to a healthy lifestyle of good nutrition and regular physical activity. The benefits of a healthy lifestyle include a greater sense of well-being, more energy and more effective living.

Achieving and Maintaining Weight Loss

Once you achieve your goals of a healthy weight, you can set new goals. Unfortunately, many people abandon their efforts because of their inability to meet unrealistic goals and expectations.

To lose weight healthfully and successfully, you can use several important tools. Review the following strategies and find ways to incorporate them into your plan:

The Importance of Physical Activity

Weight gain and obesity are often viewed as problems of eating too much. While this is part of the problem, obesity is just as likely to result from too little physical activity. Many experts feel that the alarming increase in being overweight and obese is a result of the sedentary lifestyles of most Americans. Today nearly 25 percent of Americans are completely sedentary, and up to 60 percent do not get enough physical activity to benefit their health. Increasing physical activity—energy expenditure—is as important to weight control as decreasing calorie intake.

What the Research Shows

An important study published in the *American Journal of Clinical Nutrition* surveyed nearly 800 men and women from the National Weight Control Registry who maintained an average weight loss of more than 60 pounds for over 5 years. In this survey, 90 percent of the participants reported regular physical activity as a part of their program. Other studies have reported similar findings.

A series of studies reported by researchers from the Cooper Institute for Aerobics Research in Dallas, Texas, reveal that death rates from all causes are much lower in obese men with a moderate to high level of physical fitness than in normal-weight men with low physical fitness. These important studies confirm that a lifestyle of physical activity and healthy eating is more important than the number on the scale. In other words, as the researchers from this study reported: "It's better to be fit and fat than lean and sedentary."

The Benefits of Physical Activity

- It helps the body burn fat and protects against the muscle loss associated with low-calorie eating plans.
- It helps the body maintain or increase its metabolic rate.
- It may help suppress appetite.
- It allows for weight loss on a higher calorie eating plan, which helps the body get all the nutrients it needs.
- It improves mood and self-esteem.
- It results in important health benefits such as lower blood pressure, improved cholesterol levels and increased fitness.
- It promotes long-term weight maintenance.

More Strategies for Successful Weight Loss

Keep a Record

Studies confirm that one of the most effective factors in weight loss is keeping a food and activity diary. Keeping a record is helpful for observing and evaluating your habits, moods and choices. Reviewing your records regularly can help you prepare for situations and feelings that make it difficult for you to stick with your plan. Keeping a weight chart and other important health information is also important in monitoring your progress.

Get the Support of Family and Friends

Support of family and friends helps promote success for many people. Surround yourself with people who can provide you with the positive support and encouragement you need for success.

It's also important to watch out for people who can sabotage your efforts. Do you know people who continually offer you food, encourage you to eat less healthy foods, interfere with your physical activity or find other ways to try to derail your efforts to lose weight and eat more healthy?

Take some time to consider some ways family and friends can help you reach your goals. Make a plan to ask them for the specific help you need. It's also important to identify those people who make it difficult for you to reach your goals.

Learn to Manage Your Stress

Emotional and physical stress can make it difficult to stick with a healthy lifestyle. Dealing with stress appropriately through prayer, biblical meditation, social support, relaxation exercises and other coping techniques can help you stick with your plan and achieve your goals.

Does stress influence your ability to make healthy choices and reach your goals? Read Matthew 6:25-34 and Philippians 4:4-7. Learn to give your worries to God.

Learn to Reward Yourself

Changing your lifestyle and losing weight are not easy tasks. It's important to reward yourself for your achievements. Every positive step you make—no matter how big or small—is important. Ask others to help you plan for special rewards as you reach your goals. Of course, the best rewards are those that motivate you from the inside. Learn to feel good about your accomplishments.

Do you enjoy your new lifestyle? Do you have more energy? Do you feel better? These are the best kinds of rewards. Rewards such as a new outfit or a special night out can also be helpful. Be careful not to reward yourself with too much food!

Learn to Deal With Setbacks

You *will* have setbacks and slipups. The key to successful weight loss is to see these as learning opportunities and not failures. Starting with reasonable goals and expectations is the best way to keep setbacks from becoming complete failures. Avoid absolutes such as *never, always, must* and *should*. Slipups will happen;

learn to forgive yourself and move on. Think about some situations in the past when you have allowed one slipup to knock you off your program.

understanding your eating habits

Habits are difficult to change. However, you must change your habits to achieve your goals for a healthy lifestyle. Successful change requires that you identify those habits that are keeping you from achieving your goals. It's even more important to recognize those things you're already doing that will help you achieve and maintain your goals. Most people are in such a hurry to reach their goals that they fail to make a plan they can stick with for the long haul. It's better to spend several weeks learning about yourself and making a plan than it is to jump immediately into a program that you can't stick with.

Work through the following Eating Habits Inventory to help you understand yourself and what it will take for you to reach and maintain your goals. The inventory will also help you identify those habits that you need to change. After completing the inventory, review your habits and then focus on those habits that you're most ready to change. Use it to help you develop a plan that's right for you. Review your inventory often to help you monitor your progress and adjust your plan.

Eating Habits Inventory

Understanding what foods you eat and how they influence your goals for achieving and maintaining a healthy weight will help you build a plan for successful change. Consider the following questions:

- Are you in control when it comes to eating?
- Is it easy for you to make healthy choices?
- Does stress, loneliness or an argument with a loved one cause you to overeat?
- In what situations are you most likely to lose control?
- Do you have plans to help you overcome difficult situations?
- What foods do you eat that are consistent with your goals for a healthy weight and good nutrition?
- What foods do you eat frequently that keep you from reaching your goals?
- What foods do you need to eat more often to help you reach your goals?

Now that you've thought about the foods you eat, it's important to understand that you have control over several factors that influence the choices you make, including

- What foods you buy at the grocery store
- How you plan and prepare meals at home
- The situations, people and feelings that influence the foods you eat
- What choices you make when you eat away from home (restaurants, work, social occasions, etc.)
- The variety of foods you choose to eat throughout the day

Do You

- Eat at regular times each day?
- Eat three meals each day?
- Skip meals regularly? If yes, which one(s)?
- Often wait too long between meals (six or more hours)?
- Often eat more than you want (i.e., beyond the point of being comfortably full)?
- Overeat when you're around your favorite foods?
- Often eat second helpings?
- Eat too rapidly (i.e., meals in less than 20 minutes or snacks in less than 10 minutes)?
- Eat in a place other than the dining room or at the kitchen table?
- Eat while cooking or cleaning up?
- Eat while watching television, talking on the telephone or doing other activities?

Eat Regular Meals

It's important to eat at least three regular meals each day. Your body needs fuel and a variety of nutrients throughout the day. Regular meals keep your body's tank full. Skipping meals makes it harder for you to get the nutrition you need. For example, several studies indicate that breakfast eaters are healthier and eat more nutritiously throughout the day compared to those who skip breakfast. Some experts believe that eating regular meals is also better for your body's metabolism. It's much easier to maintain your healthy habits when you stay on a regular schedule.

Healthy snacking is also an important part of an eating plan for weight loss. A regular snack can help maintain your energy levels and curb your appetite to prevent overeating at other meals. Keep your snack times consistent and have a plan for what you will eat. Keep healthy snack foods available.

Control the Amount You Eat

Slow Down!

A good way to control the amount you eat is to slow down. The slower you eat, the less likely you are to overeat and the more you'll enjoy your food. Experts estimate that it takes 20 minutes for your body to tell your brain that you've had enough to eat. Slow down and listen to your body's natural hunger signals.

Cut Down!

Continually put your knowledge of portion sizes to work for you. If you're not achieving your weight-loss goals, review your portion sizes. Serve smaller meals and don't go back for seconds unless you're truly hungry. Have a plan for when you know you will be eating your favorite foods. Limit yourself to smaller portions and eat more slowly so that you enjoy each bite. It's important to learn to stop eating when you're not hungry.

Sit Down!

It's easy to consume hidden calories if you're not paying attention to what or where you're eating. Try to have only one or two places in the house where you eat. For example, eat only while you are sitting at the dinner table. Don't eat while you're doing other activities such as cooking, watching television or talking on the telephone.

Consider Why You Overeat

Usually we eat because we're hungry. Sometimes we eat for fun and fellowship. We also eat for other reasons. Do your moods affect what you eat? If yes, which moods influence you the most?

☐ Loneliness   ☐ Anger   ☐ Fatigue   ☐ Excitement

☐ Depression   ☐ Sadness   ☐ Anxiety   ☐ Other

☐ Stress   ☐ Happiness   ☐ Boredom

Learn to avoid negative, all-or-nothing thinking: *I've blown it now; I might as well give up.* Substitute positive thoughts and activities for negative emotions. Talk to family or friends to get a better understanding of those situations and emotions that are most difficult for you. Take time to consider your emotions prayerfully.

Read, meditate on or recite encouraging and supportive Scripture. Respond to your emotions by doing other positive activities like listening to music or being physically active.

Put It All Together

Begin to make a plan for change. Focus on both your good and bad habits. For example, if you're eating lots of fruits and vegetables, that's great! Use your good habits to help you take positive steps in other areas. However, to achieve and maintain your goals for a healthy weight and good nutrition, you must focus most of your attention on those habits you need to change.

Review your Eating Inventory to better understand what factors make it difficult for you to eat healthy.

☐ My emotions often influence what I eat.   ☐ I generally eat too much.

☐ I often eat when I'm not hungry.   ☐ I eat out too much.

☐ I don't get enough physical activity.   ☐ I enjoy eating.

☐ I eat too many sweets or fattening foods.   ☐ I eat too many snacks.

☐ I don't have enough time to eat right.   ☐ I don't want to give up foods I enjoy.

Build a Plan That's Best for You

Questions to Ask Yourself
- *What habits am I most ready to change?*
- *What habits am I most confident I can change?*
- *What information, support and plans do I need to begin making these changes?*

Suggestions to Follow
- Commit yourself to a specific plan for change.
- Remember, change is best made through a series of small steps. Make sure you feel good about each step you take and reward yourself along the way.
- Review your habits and your plans regularly so that you can monitor your progress. When you experience difficulty and challenges, change your plans rather than abandoning your program.

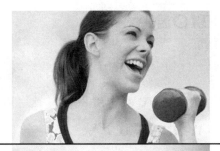

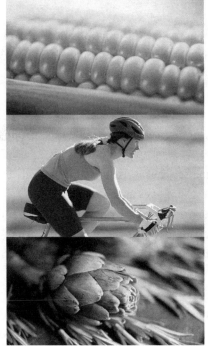

physical

WELL-BEING

dietary supplements— miracle or myth?

It seems like every time you turn around there's new information about vitamins, minerals and other supplements. If you're like most people, you may be confused about what to do! What's true and what isn't?

Sorting Through the Hype

- There are no miracle foods or supplements. Avoid anything that promises rapid results or a quick fix.
- Ignore dramatic statements that go against what most physicians, registered dietitians or national health organizations are saying.
- Stick to what you know about good nutrition, regular physical activity and a healthy lifestyle. Eating a well-balanced diet that includes a wide variety of foods is the best way to obtain the nutrients you need.
- Your best bet is to avoid anything that sounds too good to be true!

It's true—vitamins, minerals and phytochemicals are necessary for good health and provide many great benefits! However, the true benefit comes from food, not from supplements.

While we all know it's important to eat fruits and vegetables, only 20 percent of adults consume the minimum recommendation of five servings of fruits and vegetables each day. How many servings do you eat? Never substitute other foods for your exchanges of the fruits, vegetables and whole grains that you need to eat. Better yet, get lots of regular physical activity and add a few extra servings. When it comes to fruits and vegetables, studies show that eating seven or more servings a day may offer additional health benefits.

Energy in a Pill?

Not likely! Vitamins and minerals do not supply energy—that's the job of calories from carbohydrates and fats. However, vitamins and minerals are a part of the process of changing the food you eat into energy your body can use. They're also important for many chemical reactions that take place in your body every day. The best scientific evidence suggests that your body uses vitamins and minerals best in the combinations found naturally in food.

Headlines! Headlines! Read All About It!

It seems like new information about vitamins makes the news every month. You may have heard about antioxidants, homocysteine and phytochemicals. Here are some brief explanations of what medical science has discovered.

Antioxidants

Three antioxidants are most often in the headlines: beta carotene, vitamin E and vitamin C. Antioxidants help maintain healthy cells by protecting them against oxidation and the damaging effects of free radicals. Free radicals are potentially damaging oxygen molecules that are produced naturally by the body. Some experts believe that environmental factors such as smoking, air pollution and other stressors increase the production of free radicals. Studies suggest that antioxidants in fruits, vegetables and other foods may help reduce the risk of heart disease, certain cancers and a variety of other health problems. Most experts feel that more studies need to be done before specific recommendations for supplementation can be made.

Homocysteine

You may have heard about homocysteine—a protein in the blood. High levels may be associated with an increased risk of heart attack and stroke. Homocysteine levels can be influenced by what you eat. The B vitamins—folic acid, B_6 and B_{12}—help to break down homocysteine in the body. So far, there are no studies showing that taking B vitamins will lower your risk for heart attack and stroke. Everyone should follow an eating plan that has plenty of folic acid and vitamins B_6 and B_{12}. Good sources of these are citrus fruits, tomatoes, dark-green leafy vegetables and fortified cereals and grain products (rice, oats and wheat flour). Eggs, fish, chicken and lean red meats are also good sources.

Phytochemicals

Phytochemicals—plant chemicals—are substances that plants naturally produce to protect themselves against disease. These same compounds appear to have very beneficial effects on our health as well. You may have heard about some of these: isoflavones, sulphoranes, lycopene and other carotenoids to name a few. At this time, there is no evidence that these chemicals can be concentrated in pill form to provide health benefits. Take your phytochemicals in the form of fruits, vegetables and whole grains.

Questions and Answers

Do I Need to Take Supplements?

Currently none of the major health organizations such as the American Heart Association, the American Cancer Society or the American Dietetic Association recommend that healthy adults routinely take vitamin or mineral supplements for general health. There's simply not enough information on the dosages or combinations of vitamins, minerals and other nutrients that work best—or work at all!

For the time being, it is best to get the vitamins, minerals and phytochemicals your body needs from the foods you eat. Supplements simply cannot re-create what God has supplied naturally through fruits, vegetables, whole grains and other nutritious foods. Eat a variety of fruits, vegetables and whole grains each day. Balance these foods with lean meats and low-fat dairy products to get the balance and variety you need for a vitamin-packed eating plan.

What If I'm Already Taking Vitamin and Mineral Supplements?

There is no evidence that taking a multivitamin and mineral supplement that does not exceed the Recommended Daily Allowances (RDAs) is associated with any harmful effects. Vitamin and mineral supplements can be an important part of an overall health plan if taking them helps you to live a healthier lifestyle—i.e., eating a healthy diet and being more physically active. However, dietary supplements are not a substitute for eating healthy! Vitamin and mineral doses higher than the RDAs should only be taken after seeking advice from your physician or a registered dietitian. For otherwise healthy people, there is only limited data suggesting advantages for taking certain vitamin or mineral supplements in excess of the RDAs.

Are Dietary Supplements More Appropriate for Some People?

Supplements may be appropriate for some people.

- Osteoporosis, iron deficiency, digestive disorders and other health conditions may be treated or prevented with certain dietary supplements.
- People who follow very low-calorie eating plans or restrictive eating patterns (such as a vegetarian who consumes no meat or dairy foods) may need supplements. However, we do not recommend these restrictive eating plans.
- People who can't eat certain foods may need a supplement to give the body what it needs.
- Women planning to become pregnant or who are pregnant/breast-feeding should talk to their doctor about the need for certain supplements such as folic acid and iron.

the food guide pyramid*

For everything God created is good.
1 Timothy 4:4

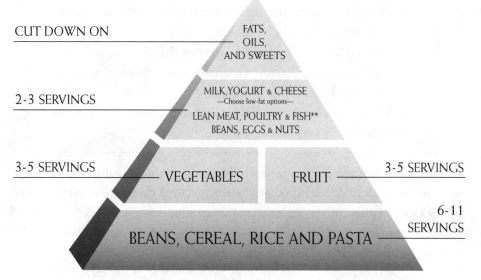

CUT DOWN ON — FATS, OILS, AND SWEETS

2-3 SERVINGS — MILK, YOGURT & CHEESE
—Choose low-fat options—
LEAN MEAT, POULTRY & FISH**
BEANS, EGGS & NUTS

3-5 SERVINGS — VEGETABLES   FRUIT — 3-5 SERVINGS

6-11 SERVINGS

BEANS, CEREAL, RICE AND PASTA —

Eat a variety of foods for good health and plenty of energy.

Adapted from United States Department of Agriculture Food Guide Pyramid

* The Food Guide Pyramid has been adapted by First Place to more closely reflect our program and recommendations.
**Note: A serving of meat, poultry or fish is two to three ounces, compared to one-ounce servings for the exchange list.

The Food Guide Pyramid, introduced in 1992 by the United States Department of Agriculture (USDA) and now adapted by most major health and nutrition organizations, offers a visual and practical way to put healthy nutrition into practice. The pyramid divides all foods into five groups based on their nutritional similarities and the number of servings needed for a healthy diet (much like exchanges). It includes an additional category for fats, oils and sweets, which should be eaten sparingly. Each food group supplies some, but not all, of the nutrients you need. No one food or food group is more important than another; you need them all for nutritional health. By eating a variety of foods from each group, sticking with the recommended number of servings and putting into practice the principles of portion control, you will be better able to achieve your goals for healthy weight and good health.

Determining the Number of Servings

The pyramid shows a range of servings for each major food group. The number of servings that are right for you depends on how many calories you need, which in turn depends on your age, sex, size and how active you are. Almost everyone should have at least the lowest number of servings in each range.

For Adults and Teens
- 1,600 calories are about right for many sedentary women and some older adults.
- 2,200 calories are about right for most children, teenage girls, active women and many sedentary men. Women who are pregnant or breast-feeding may need more calories.
- 2,800 calories are about right for teenage boys, many active men and some very active women.

Take a look at the following table that tells you how many servings you need for your calorie level. If you are between calorie categories, you will estimate servings within the ranges indicated. For example, some less active women may need only 2,000 calories to maintain a healthy weight. For a 2,000-calorie level, eight servings from the bread/grain group would be about right.

Food Groups	1,600 Calories	2,200 Calories	2,800 Calories
Bread/Grain Servings	6	9	11
Vegetable Servings	3	4	5
Fruit Servings	2	3	4
Milk Servings	2-3[1]	2-3[1]	2-3[1]
Meat Group[2] (in ounces)	5	6	7

1. Women who are pregnant or breast-feeding, teenagers and young adults up to age 24 need 3 servings.
2. Meat group amounts are in total ounces.

If You Want to Lose Weight

The best and simplest way to lose weight is to increase your physical activity and reduce the fat and sugars in your diet. But be sure to eat at least the lowest number of suggested servings from each of the five major food groups in the Food Guide Pyramid. You need them for the vitamins, minerals, carbohydrates and protein they provide. For best results, try to pick the lowest fat choices from each of the food groups.

For more information on the Food Guide Pyramid, check the
USDA website at www.nal.usda.gov/fnic/Fpyr/pyramid.html.

choosing high-fiber foods

Many of the foods you eat influence your risk for several diseases, including heart disease, stroke, diabetes and certain cancers. Following an eating plan that is high in fiber and low in saturated fat and cholesterol reduces your risk for these diseases. High-fiber foods may also help you achieve and maintain a healthy weight. Health experts recommend that you eat 25 to 30 grams of fiber each day; the national average is 15 or fewer grams!

You can get all the fiber you need if you eat a variety of foods, including:

- Six to 11 servings of bread, cereal, rice, pasta and other grains daily. At least three servings from this group should include whole-grain foods.
- Five or more servings of fruits and vegetables daily.
- Legumes—beans, peas, soybeans and lentils—at least once or twice each week.

Fiber Facts

Fiber is found only in the cell walls of plants—fruits, vegetables and grains. Your body does not digest or absorb fiber. Grains are made up of three parts—bran, endosperm and germ. Most processed grain foods are made from the endosperm. The endosperm contains the energy—carbohydrates and protein—but little of the fiber, vitamins, minerals and phytochemicals (plant chemicals believed to promote health). Whole grains also contain the bran and the germ, which are higher in fiber and nutrients. There are two main types of fiber in the diet—soluble and insoluble.

Soluble fiber dissolves in water and forms a gel in the digestive system. The texture of foods like cooked oatmeal comes from soluble fiber. Soluble fiber lowers blood cholesterol levels by blocking the absorption of cholesterol and fats from the diet. It may also have other cholesterol-lowering effects. In fact, scientists have isolated a component of soluble fiber called beta-glucan that appears to be responsible for many of these benefits. Soluble fiber may also help lower blood sugar. Good sources of soluble fiber include oatmeal, oat bran, barley, dried beans, peas, brown rice and apples.

Insoluble fiber does not dissolve in water. Insoluble fiber is more important in digestive health. It provides the roughage that improves bowel function and lowers your risk of colon cancer. Except for being a substitute for foods higher in fat and cholesterol, insoluble fiber does not appear to lower cholesterol levels. Good sources of insoluble fiber are whole-grain breads and cereals, wheat bran and most fruits and vegetables.

Dietary Fiber and Weight Control

Both types of fiber may help in weight control. High-fiber foods are more filling and less fattening (i.e., they are usually lower in calories and fat). Also, eating meals that are high in fiber—fruits, vegetables, whole grains and legumes—leaves less room for foods that are high in calories and fat. Very high fiber, low-calorie diets are not good ways to lose weight because they come up short in other important nutrients. Fiber supplements are also not recommended for weight loss. Balance, moderation and variety are the keys to good nutrition!

Getting Enough of the Right Kind of Fiber

Do you eat three servings of whole grains each day? Experts recommend that at least 3 of the 6 to 11 servings of breads, cereals, rice and pasta that you eat every day be whole grains. White and wheat breads, white rice, refined pasta and many cereals do not count as whole grain. Look for "whole grain," "multigrain" or "whole wheat" on the label. Don't let the names "wheat bread" and "wheat cereal" fool you—these foods are often colored with caramel or molasses. Look at the label—does it contain 2 or more grams of fiber per serving?

What foods can you add to your eating plan to boost your intake of fiber? Eating at least five servings of fruits and vegetables and six servings of breads, cereals, rice, pasta and other grains each day should give you most of the fiber you need each day. For extra insurance, make sure that you're choosing several foods that are high in fiber. The following table will help you make healthful choices:

Food	Serving	Fiber (in grams)	Soluble	Insoluble
White bread	1 slice	Less than 1		
Wheat bread	1 slice	Less than 1		
White rice	½ cup	Less than 1		
Refined pasta	½ cup	Less than 1		
Graham crackers	2 squares	2		✓
Broccoli	½ cup	2		✓
Orange	1 medium	2		✓
Whole wheat bread	1 slice	2 to 3		✓
Whole-grain bread	1 slice	2 to 3		✓
Whole wheat pasta	½ cup	2 to 3		✓
Bran muffin	1 medium	2 to 3	✓	✓
Oat, oatmeal	¾ cup	3	✓	✓
Apple with skin	1 medium	3	✓	✓
Brown rice	½ cup	3 to 4	✓	✓
Potato with skin	1 medium	3 to 4	✓	✓
Legumes and peas	½ cup	4 to 6	✓	✓
Bran cereal	½ cup	6 to 15	✓	✓

Increasing the Fiber in Your Diet

- Choose more whole- or multigrain breads. Look for whole wheat or whole-grain flour as the first ingredient.
- Start your day with a bowl of whole-grain or bran cereal.
- Try adding $\frac{1}{4}$ cup of wheat bran to foods such as cereal, pancakes, applesauce, yogurt or meat loaf.
- When baking, substitute whole wheat flour for half of the white flour called for in the recipe.
- In baked goods, substitute oats for one-third of the flour called for in the recipe.
- Mix at least one-half refined pasta or white rice with whole-grain pasta or brown rice in dishes.
- Increase your intake of beans, lentils, soybeans and peas. Use them instead of meat in casseroles or other dishes.
- Add legumes, wheat bran or other grains to soups, pasta, salads and other dishes.
- Leave the skin on fruits and vegetables such as apples, pears, peaches and potatoes.
- Add fresh or dried fruits to cereals and salads.
- Add extra vegetables to salads, soups and other dishes.
- Read food labels. Foods with more than 2.5 grams of fiber per serving are good sources of fiber.

off to a good start

Breakfast may be the most important meal of the day. After all, your body hasn't had any food for 8 to 12 hours—it's time to break the fast. After a night's sleep, your body needs a fresh supply of fuel and nutrients to start the day. Your mind needs energy to be sharp. Your muscles need energy to keep you on the move. A healthy breakfast gives your body what it needs.

Research Results

- Several studies show that breakfast eaters perform better mentally and physically.
- Some studies suggest that breakfast skippers are more likely to overeat later in the day. Approaching snack time or lunch on an empty stomach can lead to poor choices and overeating.
- Studies show that regular breakfast eaters consume more nutrients throughout the day. Regular breakfast eaters are more likely to get adequate levels of minerals, such as calcium, phosphorus and magnesium, and vitamins, such as riboflavin, folate and vitamins A, C and B_{12}.
- One study of nearly 3,500 men and women found that regular cereal eaters eat less fat during the day, have a lower cholesterol intake and eat more fiber. They also have lower blood cholesterol levels. All these factors add up to a lower risk for heart disease.

Unfortunately, despite all the benefits of starting the day with a healthy breakfast, it's the meal most often skipped.

Healthy Choices

While eating any kind of breakfast may be better than skipping, it's important to make healthy choices. Soft drinks, sugary cereals, pastries, fried potatoes and high-fat meats are not a healthy way to go. These foods supply calories your body needs for energy but can be high in fat, cholesterol and sugar and low in vitamins, minerals and fiber. A balanced breakfast will give you the sustained energy and nutrients your body needs.

Try to eat a well-balanced breakfast high in complex carbohydrates, some protein and a little fat. Whole-grain cereals and breads, nonfat milk, yogurt, fruit and even eggs are good choices. These foods stay with you longer and give you the energy you need to make it through the morning. Many breakfast foods are high in simple sugars and can quickly leave you feeling hungry again.

Cereal

Hot and cold cereals are a great start to any day. Fortified cereals provide vitamins, such as folate and other B vitamins, and minerals, such as iron and calcium. Adding low-fat milk boosts the protein, B vitamins and minerals such as calcium, phosphorus and magnesium. High-fiber cereals help keep your digestive system working regularly and provide other important health benefits.

Balance out your breakfast and get a start on your five-a-day goal by eating fresh fruit with your cereal.

Read the Nutrition Facts panel and the ingredient list to find the cereals best for you. Look for high-fiber, low-sugar and vitamin-fortified brands. You want the first ingredients listed to be whole grains or rolled oats. Look for cereals with 5 to 10 grams (or fewer) of sugar and more than 2.5 grams of fiber per serving. Low-fat cereals have no more than 2 to 3 grams of fat. Watch out for granola because it is often high in fat and sugar. Some varieties of cereal are fortified with 100 percent of the Recommended Daily Intake for vitamins and minerals—just make sure to finish the milk in the bottom of the bowl!

Creative Solutions

What are some creative and enjoyable ways you can begin to make a healthy breakfast part of your daily routine? Try the following tips to help get you started:

- Make sure you wake up in time to fit in a good breakfast—10 to 15 minutes is all you need. To save time, prepare for breakfast before you go to bed.
- If you don't have time to eat at home or if you're not hungry first thing in the morning, drink a small glass of low-fat milk, or fruit or vegetable juice on the way to work. You can pack a bagel, breakfast bar, yogurt, peanut-butter sandwich, cheese and crackers or fresh fruit to eat on the way to or at work.
- Make eating breakfast a family affair. Start the day connecting with your family and fueling your bodies for the day ahead. What a great time to start the day with prayer!
- It takes just minutes to make a delicious smoothie. Simply mix nonfat yogurt, frozen fruit and juice or milk in a blender—experiment! Drink it while you're getting ready for or on your way to work.
- Pop frozen waffles (preferably whole grain) into the toaster and top with jam, jelly, yogurt, low-fat cream cheese or peanut butter. You can do the same with whole-grain breads, bagels or English muffins.
- Skip the fat-laden breakfast sandwiches offered by fast-food chains. Make your own from low-fat cheese, lean ham or turkey, bread, bagel or an English muffin.

- Who says you have to eat a traditional breakfast in the morning? Leftover vegetable pizza, grilled-cheese sandwiches, burritos and other lunch and dinnertime favorites are options you can choose. You can have a quick and nutritious breakfast by reheating leftovers.

Breakfast in the Fast Lane

Do you find yourself eating breakfast away from home or in the car? The following tips will help you make healthy choices:

- Hot and cold cereals are a good choice at any restaurant.
- Pancakes and waffles can be a good choice if you go easy on the butter or margarine. Top them with fresh fruit, jam, jelly or syrup.
- Order fruit juice and low-fat milk instead of coffee or a soft drink.
- Eggs are a good choice because they are a good source of protein, iron and vitamin A. It's the egg yolks that are high in cholesterol; ask for scrambled eggs without the yolk or made with an egg substitute.
- A bagel or English muffin is a good choice, but watch the butter and cream cheese. Most muffins are high in fat and calories, as are pastries, croissants and biscuits.

outsmarting the snack attack

If you want to lose weight, you've got to cut out the snacks!

Have you heard that before? Actually, it's not the snacking that's bad, it's the usual snack choices—chips, crackers, dips, cookies, candy bars, etc.—that are the problem. The truth is that your body works best when it refuels every four to six hours. The best way to fuel your body is to eat light, well-balanced meals and two or three healthy snacks. Snacking may even help you lose weight by taming your appetite, thus preventing the tendency to overeat and make poor choices. Learn to make healthy snacks a part of your daily eating plan.

Snack Facts

Surveys suggest that 99 percent of Americans snack, and 75 percent do so one or more times each day. How much do we spend on snacking? Over $40 million each day. Snacking accounts for nearly 25 percent of daily calories, and by the end of one year the average person has consumed over 22 pounds of snack foods, mostly chips, pretzels, puffs and candy. On the positive side, many of our favorite snack foods now come in low-fat versions. On the down side, many of these are still high in calories and low in nutrition. Why do you snack?

- ☐ To satisfy hunger
- ☐ To satisfy cravings
- ☐ To fight boredom and pass time
- ☐ To boost energy
- ☐ To relax
- ☐ For enjoyment and pleasure
- ☐ For nourishment
- ☐ For emotional comfort

It's important to understand the reasons why you snack. It's also important to know how your typical snack foods stack up nutritionally. Use snacks to satisfy hunger, nourish your body, boost your energy and help you reach your goals for a healthy weight.

Healthy Snacking

The key to healthy nutrition is variety, balance and moderation. With these principles in mind, snacking can be an important part of a healthy eating plan. Snack time can be a great way to get in your daily servings of fruits, vegetables and whole grains. Low-fat dairy foods such as milk and yogurt also make healthy snacks. Keep a supply of healthy snacks in convenient locations. Concentrate on complex carbohydrates and low-fat proteins. Do whatever you can to avoid those high-fat, high-sugar treats that always seem to show up at home, work and social occasions. Healthy beverages can also be great at snack time; water, fruit or vegetable juice, and low-fat milk are your best choices.

The important thing to remember about snacking is that *when* you eat is not as important as *what* and *how much* you eat. When it comes to weight control the issue is total calories—not when or how often you eat. As for snacking, eat only when you're hungry and stop when you're full!

How Snacks Stack Up

Snacks	Calories	Fat
Ice cream (1 cup)	~ 300	~ 15 grams
Candy Bar (2 ounces)	~ 250	~ 12 grams
Mixed nuts (1 ounce or 20 nuts)	~ 200	~ 15 grams
Fried chips (1 ounce or 10 chips)	~ 160	~ 10 grams
Microwave popcorn (3 cups)	~ 150	~ 10 grams
Nonfat fruit yogurt (1 cup)	~ 120	0
Baked chips (1 ounce or 13 chips)	~ 110	~ 1 gram
Pretzels (1 ounce or 9 pretzels)	~ 110	~ 1 gram
Fresh fruit (1 medium)	~ 60	trace
Air-popped popcorn (3 cups)	~ 50	trace
Vegetable (1/2 cup)	~ 25	trace

Plan Ahead

Stock your home, office and workout bag with a variety of healthy snacks so you'll always have something healthy on hand when hunger strikes. Buy several plastic containers, plastic bags, a thermos and an insulated lunch bag or cooler to make it easy for you to carry snacks with you. Keep a special shopping list to help you remember to stock up on healthy snack foods. Instead of looking for low-fat versions of your favorite processed snack foods, choose foods such as whole-grain breads and crackers, fruits, vegetables, rice cakes and low-fat yogurt.

healthy snack choices

50-Calorie Snacks	Exchanges
30 small pretzel sticks	1 bread
1 tangerine	½ fruit
2 tomatoes	2 fruits
1 cup zucchini sticks	1 vegetable
1 large dill pickle	½ vegetable
1 (4-inch) rice cake	½ bread
1 cup tomato juice	1½ vegetables
1 carrot	1½ vegetables
2 gingersnaps	½ bread, ½ fat
¾ cup raspberries	1 fruit
12 strawberries	½ fruit
½ cup fat-free milk	½ milk
8 celery ribs	2 vegetables
4 saltine crackers	½ bread, ½ fat
2 fortune cookies	1 bread (sugar)
2 cups broccoli florets	2 vegetables
1 kiwi fruit	1 fruit
3 apricots	1 fruit
½ cup blueberries	½ fruit
10 ripe olives	1 fat
½ cup orange juice	1 fruit
1 medium cucumber	2 vegetables
4 slices melba toast	½ bread
1 medium peach	½ fruit
1 cup strawberries	½ fruit
6 cherry tomatoes	1 vegetable
¾ cup consommé or broth	½ meat
12 whole radishes	½ vegetable
1 caramel popcorn cake	1 bread
2 slices garlic crisp bread	½ bread
½ cup mandarin orange slices	½ fruit
¼ cup tropical fruit salad	½ fruit

sweetness by any other name

Many different sugars are found naturally in foods. Sugars are also added in the preparation and manufacturing of many foods. In addition to tasting good, sugar plays several important roles in food. It gives certain foods their characteristic texture, color and consistency. You may have discovered the difference sugar makes when you reduce or substitute it in recipes.

Myths and misinformation about sugar and other sweeteners are very common. Common table sugar, or refined sugar, tops the misinformation list. You've probably also heard stories about saccharin and aspartame. Whether the sugar comes from the sugar bowl, honey, fruit, vegetables or milk, there's little difference from your body's viewpoint. In the end, your body converts sugars and starches from fruits, vegetables, grains and other foods to glucose. Along with fatty acids (fat), glucose is the main energy source for your body.

The Truth About Sugar

A gram of sugar contains four calories. That's less than half of the nine calories supplied by a gram of fat. A teaspoon of sugar contains 16 calories. A soft drink can have 9 to 12 teaspoons of sugar! What's the real problem? The estimated 150 pounds of sugar that the average American consumes each year add up to a lot of calories. The bottom line is that too many calories are fattening, and it doesn't really matter whether the extra calories come from sugars, fat or protein. We gain weight when we take in more calories from our food than we expend in physical activity. The problem with sugar is that it often supplies empty calories (i.e., calories without the nutrition). Sugar is also often found in foods that are high in calories and fat. Because most of us have a sweet tooth, sugary foods often replace other more nutritious foods in our diets.

What's in a Name?

Acesulfame K	Glucose	Maple syrup
Aspartame	High-fructose corn syrup	Molasses
Brown sugar	Honey	Saccharin
Corn sweeteners	Lactose	Sorbitol
Dextrose	Maltose	Sugar
Fruit-juice concentrate	Mannitol	Xylitol

While there are some minor differences, your body treats these sugars much the same. In terms of nutritional value there's virtually no difference. The nonnutritive sweeteners—acesulfame K, aspartame and saccharin—add sweetness without the calories.

How Sweet It Is!

Nonnutritive sweeteners (also known as artificial, or intense, sweeteners) can give you the taste of sugar without the calories. It's important to read product labels; many foods labeled "sugar free" contain a sugar substitute, or nonnutritive sweetener. Even though foods made with nonnutritive sweeteners may be low in calories, many of them may also be low in nutrition. In a healthy eating plan, calories are not the only issue—you need to consider nutrition (i.e., vitamins, minerals, phytochemicals and fiber).

Four artificial sweeteners are commonly used today: aspartame, acesulfame potassium, saccharin and sucralose.

- **Aspartame** (e.g., NutraSweet and Equal) is a newer nonnutritive sweetener that actually contains calories. Because it's 180 times as sweet as sugar, you need only a tiny amount to sweeten food. It's actually a combination of two amino acids. One problem with aspartame is that it loses its sweetness when heated. Consequently, you cannot use it in baked goods, such as cakes. You can use it in top-of-the-stove foods like pudding by adding it at the very end of cooking. Available scientific evidence does not support various health concerns reported by some individuals.
- **Acesulfame potassium** (e.g., Sunett) is 200 times sweeter than sugar and was first approved in 1988 as a tabletop sweetener. It is now approved for products such as baked goods, frozen desserts, candies and beverages. More than 90 studies verify its safety. It is often combined with other sweeteners. Worldwide, the sweetener is used in more than 4,000 products, according to its manufacturer, Nutrinova. It has excellent shelf life and does not break down when cooked or baked.
- **Saccharin** (e.g., Sweet'n Low) has been around for over 100 years. It's over 300 times sweeter than table sugar—a little goes a long way! Saccharin can be used in both hot and cold foods to make them sweeter. Substituting saccharin for sugar in baked goods may change their taste, texture and appearance. The risk of cancer associated with

the use of saccharin in laboratory animals appears to be very low or nonexistent in humans.

- **Sucralose** (e.g., Splenda) is 600 times sweeter than sugar. It was approved in 1998 as a tabletop sweetener and for use in products such as baked goods, beverages, gum, frozen dairy desserts, fruit juices and gelatins. It is now approved as a general-purpose sweetener for all foods. It is bulked up with maltodextrin, a starchy powder, so it will measure more like sugar. It has a good shelf life and doesn't degrade when exposed to heat.

The key with both sugars and nonnutritive sweeteners is moderation. Let your overall goals of achieving and maintaining a healthy weight and good health help you decide what is best for you.

The Wise Use of Sugar

Moderation, balance and variety are the keys to achieving and maintaining a healthy weight and good nutrition. Some dietitians actually advise people trying to lose weight to include some sugary foods in their diets. Eating plans that restrict certain foods are often too hard to maintain. Trying to eliminate certain foods often leads to an eventual slipup (i.e., you break down and eat that food). Slipups often lead to feelings of guilt and failure. The feelings cause many people to abandon their weight-loss efforts. Others report that there are certain foods they need to avoid in order to achieve their goals. If eating some sugary foods allows you to better reach your goals, that's okay. If eliminating sugary foods or using nonnutritive sweeteners helps you reach your goals, that's okay too! You must decide what's best for you and your body.

There are no good or bad foods, only bad diets. Your eating plan should not focus on what you're eliminating but what you're adding—good nutrition, improved health and a higher quality of life.

the truth about fats

"Low fat," "fat free," "nonfat," "no fat," "less fat," "reduced fat"—too much fat! Surveys reveal that dietary fat is the number-one nutritional concern of Americans. In fact, reducing dietary fat has become an obsession for many. Despite our knowledge about fat and the availability of more low-fat foods, the number of Americans who are overweight or obese is on the rise.

Fats Are Essential for Good Health!
Fats are an important source of energy. They supply, carry and store the fat-soluble vitamins—A, D, E and K. Fats are involved in the production of nerve cells, cell membranes and many important hormones. Fat helps your body maintain healthy skin and hair. Body fat cushions and insulates the body. Fat also gives certain foods their taste, texture and aroma. Fat satisfies hunger and makes many foods more pleasurable to eat. However, too much fat in the diet is associated with heart disease, certain cancers, diabetes, obesity and high blood pressure.

How Much Fat Do I Need?
With fat intake averaging about 34 percent of calories, the typical American diet is still too high in fat. The goal is to keep total fat intake to 30 percent or less calories. Fat contains 9 calories per gram, which is over twice the calories supplied by carbohydrates and proteins. Because high-fat foods contain more calories, they probably increase the likelihood of weight gain. However, too many calories and not enough physical activity are the real problems. Even eating low-fat foods high in calories will result in weight gain.

Variety, balance and moderation are the keys to a healthy eating plan. Cutting fat without cutting calories or without getting more physical activity will not help you lose weight.

Different Types of Fat
All fats are made up of carbon, hydrogen and oxygen molecules and are classified by their chemical structure—saturated, polyunsaturated and monounsaturated. Most foods contain all three types of fats but in different amounts.

Saturated

- Saturated fats have all the hydrogen molecules they can hold. This saturation with hydrogen creates a rigid structure that is solid at room temperature.
- Saturated fats raise blood cholesterol levels more than any other type of fat. Animal foods such as meat, poultry, fish, butter, milk and cheese are high in saturated fats. Coconut oil, palm oil and palm kernel oil are also high in saturated fat.

Polyunsaturated and Monounsaturated

- Polyunsaturated and monounsaturated fats are not saturated with hydrogen molecules. Because they are unsaturated, they have flexible structures that are fluid at room temperature. Vegetable oils are higher in unsaturated fats.
- Polyunsaturated fats may help decrease blood cholesterol levels when substituted for saturated fats. Common sources of polyunsaturated fats are safflower oil, sunflower oil, corn oil, soybean oil and many nuts and seeds.
- Monounsaturated fats also help decrease blood cholesterol levels when substituted for saturated fats. Common sources of monounsaturated fats are olive oil, canola oil, peanut oil and avocados.

Cutting Down Fat

When it comes to calories, all fats are created equal. Because all fats are high in calories, cutting back on fat can help you consume fewer calories and lose weight—physical activity helps, too! The highest sources of dietary fat are found in meats, cheese, eggs, dairy products, desserts, snack foods and nuts. The key to low-fat eating is learning to choose the foods highest in nutrition and lowest in calories—whole grains, fruits, vegetables, lean meats, poultry, fish and low-fat dairy products. Much of the fat in our diet is added—butter, margarine, cheese, oils and salad dressings. Use less of these fats in cooking and preparation. Also, make the switch to low-fat or nonfat alternatives when available. But remember, not all low-fat versions of cakes, cookies or snack foods are low calorie!

Eat Less Saturated Fat

Saturated fat is the main culprit when it comes to high blood cholesterol levels. Specifically, eating lots of saturated fat will increase the LDL cholesterol, which is the bad cholesterol that's linked to fatty buildup in the arteries. Certain cancers may also be related to higher intakes of saturated fat. That's why it's especially important to limit intake of this type of fat.

Meat is where Americans get most of the saturated fat and cholesterol in their diet—although cheese is a close second. Instead of fatty meats, look for lean cuts of beef and pork, usually labeled "loin" or "round." And look for lean or extra-lean ground beef, chicken or turkey. Buy cuts labeled "select" rather than "prime" or "choice." Remove extra fat and use low-fat cooking methods—grill, boil, broil, bake and roast instead of frying. Look for reduced-fat or fat-free versions of luncheon meats and hot dogs.

More Useful Tips

- Use all fats and oils sparingly, selecting polyunsaturated and monounsaturated fats instead of saturated fats such as butter, lard, shortening and tropical oils (coconut, palm and palm kernel).
- Drink nonfat or low-fat milk (1%) and choose low-fat or nonfat versions of yogurt and sour cream.
- Learn to modify your recipes with low-fat substitutions.
- Limit the amount of cheese in your eating plan. Choose cheeses with 3 to 5 grams of fat per ounce. Use $\frac{1}{3}$ to $\frac{1}{2}$ less cheese than a recipe calls for. You can even mix low-fat and nonfat versions to cut down on fat and calories. Ounce for ounce, cheese is as high in fat and saturated fat as meat!
- Choose low-fat salad dressings and mayonnaise with no more than 1 gram of saturated fat per tablespoon. Choose mustard, ketchup and other low-fat spreads and condiments more often.
- Limit the number of eggs you eat each week to two or three. Or substitute two egg whites for every whole egg—the yolks contain most of the fat and cholesterol—or use cholesterol-free egg substitutes.
- Use low-fat cooking methods: Make low-fat substitutions in your recipes; sauté using low-sodium broth instead of oils and other fats; chill soups and stews and skim off the fat that collects on the surface.
- Cut down on bakery and snack foods—cakes, cookies, pastries, doughnuts and chips. Even low-fat versions can be high in calories!

Note: Children below the age of two should not
follow a fat-restricted diet.

All Fats Are Not Created Equal

In terms of calories, all fats add up to 9 calories per gram. However, not all fats are created equal when it comes to health, so it's important to pay attention to the types of fat you eat. Specific fats have different effects on cholesterol levels and other aspects of your overall health. You're probably aware that diets high in saturated fat and cholesterol are associated with higher levels of blood cholesterol and greater risk for heart disease and certain cancers. Specific fats—in moderation—may even have beneficial effects on health. Monounsaturated fatty acids in olive and canola oils may increase HDL (*good*) cholesterol in some people when substituted for saturated fat in the diet.

No one is recommending that you increase the amount of fat in your eating plan, but it is important to shift the balance in favor of healthier choices. Experts recommend the following limitations:

- Total fat to 30 percent or less of calories.
- Saturated fat to less than 10 percent of calories.
- Polyunsaturated fat to 10 percent of calories.
- Monounsaturated fat to between 10 percent and 15 percent of calories.

Rating the Oils

Fats and oils contain a combination of all three types of fatty acids: saturated, polyunsaturated and monounsaturated. All oils are 100 percent fat and contain 120 calories per tablespoon. The following chart compares fats higher in unsaturated fatty acids with those higher in saturated fatty acids.

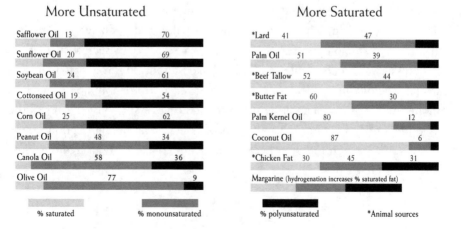

More Unsaturated

Safflower Oil	13	70
Sunflower Oil	20	69
Soybean Oil	24	61
Cottonseed Oil	19	54
Corn Oil	25	62
Peanut Oil	48	34
Canola Oil	58	36
Olive Oil	77	9

More Saturated

Oil		
*Lard	41	47
Palm Oil	51	39
*Beef Tallow	52	44
*Butter Fat	60	30
Palm Kernel Oil	80	12
Coconut Oil	87	6
*Chicken Fat	30	45	31
Margarine (hydrogenation increases % saturated fat)		

% saturated   % monounsaturated   % polyunsaturated   *Animal sources

The following are tips for including fats and oils in a healthy eating plan:

- Cut down on all fats and oils.
- Choose unsaturated sources of fat more often than saturated sources.
- Choose a monounsaturated source such as canola or olive oil and a polyunsaturated source such as safflower or corn oil. Use limited amounts of both in cooking and preparing foods.
- Choose soft-tub margarine with liquid vegetable oil or water listed as the first ingredient more often than margarine (with hydrogenated fats as the first ingredient), stick margarine or butter.

Fat Servings

To meet the above guidelines for total fat intake and balance, limit yourself to 3 to 5 servings of fat each day. Choose the following unsaturated fats instead of ones higher in saturated fat. One exchange equals

1 teaspoon vegetable oil	2 to 3 teaspoons seeds or nuts
1 tablespoon reduced-fat margarine	$\frac{1}{8}$ medium avocado
1 tablespoon low-fat salad dressing	1 teaspoon peanut butter
1 teaspoon regular mayonnaise	1 teaspoon regular margarine
1 tablespoon low-fat mayonnaise	5 large or 10 small olives

Hydrogenated Fats and Trans Fatty Acids

You may have heard about hydrogenated fats. Hydrogenation is a process that makes unsaturated oils more solid at room temperature (i.e., more like saturated fats). Hydrogenation also increases the amount of trans fatty acids. Trans fatty acid simply refers to where the hydrogen is placed on the fat molecule. Actually, trans fatty acids are also found naturally in many foods such as meat, butter and milk. You will commonly see the terms "partially hydrogenated" or "hydro-genated" vegetable oil on the label of many processed foods such as margarine, salad dressings, crackers, chips and other baked goods. Hydrogenated fats and trans fatty acids can raise blood cholesterol levels but probably not as much as saturated fats. Choose margarine that lists liquid vegetable oil or water as the first ingredient and no more than 2 grams of saturated fat per tablespoon. There is no reason to switch to butter because of health concerns about hydrogenated fats or trans fatty acids.

Omega-3 Fatty Acids

Omega-3 fatty acids are polyunsaturated fatty acids found mostly in cold-water fish and some vegetable oils. Omega-3 fatty acids may reduce the risk of heart disease through effects on cholesterol, blood-clotting factors and blood pressure. Good sources include salmon, albacore tuna, mackerel, sardines and lake trout. *Eat more fish!* A healthy eating plan can include several servings each week. Canola, soybean and flaxseed oils are also good sources of omega-3 fatty acids.

Fat Replacers—Fake Fats

Fat replacers are added to cheeses, desserts, salad dressings and snack foods to give them the taste and feel of the full-fat versions—without the calories! Olestra (OLEAN) is one of the newer fat replacers. It is made from a combination of vegetable fat and carbohydrate. It's calorie free because it passes through the body without being digested. Olestra appears to be safe; *however, it is known to interfere with the absorption of the fat-soluble vitamins and cause digestive discomfort in some people.*

Simplesse is a fat replacer found mostly in frozen dairy products. It's made from protein. Although foods made with fat replacers are low in fat, they still have calories and can be low in nutrients.

*As always, moderation, balance and variety are the keys
to a healthy eating plan.*

understanding fad diets

Lose Weight Without Exercising!
Take Off Pounds While You Sleep!
Lose 30 Pounds in 30 Days!
Zap 3 Inches from Your Thighs!

Doesn't it seem like everywhere you turn there's a new miracle diet or supplement being advertised or reported in the media? One of the biggest reasons people give for not starting or sticking with a healthy eating plan is confusion and frustration over all the conflicting information.

It is estimated that Americans spend over $40 billion each year on products and plans to lose weight. Despite all the money people spend, less than 20 percent are successful in losing weight over the long term.

Your Dieting History

Have you ever tried a diet or supplement that promised more than it could deliver? If you answered yes, what diets or products have you tried? Why didn't these programs or products work for you?

It's important to realize that no diet, pill or product can produce the benefits that come with following God's plan for healthy living. You are truly "fearfully and wonderfully made" (Psalm 139:14). The secret to good health and effective living is deciding to care for your body as God's good creation (see 1 Corinthians 6:19-20). Are you ready to commit to a healthy lifestyle of good nutrition and regular physical activity?

Plan Evolution

Remember, no food, diet or product provides all the magic answers for good health or weight loss. To help you sort through the confusion, use the following checklist when evaluating information:

- ☐ Does the program promise a quick fix?
- ☐ Do the claims sound too good to be true; are the words "breakthrough" or "miracle" used to describe it?
- ☐ Does the program recommend regular physical activity?
- ☐ Are only certain foods or products emphasized? Are other foods off-limits?

☐ Do you have to buy special supplements or products?

☐ Can you follow the program for a lifetime?

☐ Does the program go against the recommendation of major nutrition, medical and scientific organizations?

The Facts About Fad Diets

Most fad diets are recycled every few years with a few new twists added to make them seem different. Fad diets are usually unbalanced and don't provide the variety you need for good health or enjoyable eating.

A calorie is a calorie, whether it comes from fat, protein or carbohydrate. You gain weight when you take in more calories than your body needs. Here are some common types of fad diets to watch for.

Instant Success Through Miracle Supplements

Many fad diets take advantage of people's desire for instant results by creating the myth that certain foods or supplements have special physiologic or metabolic properties for quick weight loss. There are no known miracle foods or supplements that burn fat or promote long-term weight loss.

A weight loss of one to two pounds per week is all that the body can healthfully lose. More rapid weight loss is the result of water loss, not fat loss. Over the long term some of these diets will even result in muscle loss—especially if physical activity is not involved.

Combining Foods to Boost Metabolism

Some fad diets suggest that eating foods in certain combinations will help you burn fat more effectively, boost your metabolism or improve your health. These diets, like the ones that promote miracle foods, don't work! God did not design your body in a way that makes eating a complicated affair.

Digestion is an amazing process that uses specific enzymes in specific areas of your digestive tract. Combinations of certain foods, timing of meals or special supplements do not have any effect on this process. Another problem with these diets is that they don't provide the variety and balance your body needs for good health.

Weight Loss Without Exercise

Most fad diets don't encourage physical activity. In fact, some programs promise weight loss while you sleep! Physical activity should be one of the highest priorities of any weight-loss program. Few people can maintain long-term weight loss without regular physical activity. Besides that, we need physical activity to keep healthy and prevent disease.

Guaranteed to Work for Everyone

Avoid diets that offer a one-size-fits-all approach. There is no one diet that works for everyone. Weight regulation is a complex process that involves many factors. A good weight-loss program considers individual needs and differences. A good program allows you to personalize your eating plan. You are more likely to stick to a plan that most closely reflects your lifestyle, tastes and preferences.

Over-the-Counter Products

Fad diets may offer easy access to over-the-counter weight-loss drugs or supplements. Studies show that even approved weight-loss medications result in a weight loss of only 10 to 15 percent; it's unlikely that a product advertised in the back of a magazine or on the side of the road will be any more effective.

Some of these supplements may even cause serious side effects—even death! Never take medication or a supplement without talking to your primary doctor.

Packaged Program Foods

Many diet programs sell packaged foods. These products may make a lot of money for the commercial programs, but they may not be the most effective way to teach people how to develop and follow a healthy eating plan. To be effective, a weight-loss program must teach people how to develop lifelong habits of healthy eating and regular physical activity. This includes learning how to choose and prepare healthy foods.

"Experts" and Celebrity Endorsements

Many programs are sold by self-proclaimed experts. These experts make sensational claims and are promoted using personal success stories of famous television, film or sports celebrities.

The most reliable spokespersons have training in nutrition and medicine from reputable universities. Contact groups such as the American Dietetics Association, the American Heart Association and the American Medical Association to see if the program or product is supported by major nutrition, medical and scientific organizations. Registered dietitians (RDs) are also a good source of nutrition information.

understanding vitamins and minerals

When it comes to vitamins and minerals, does it seem that information is changing faster than you can keep up with it? If you're like most people, you probably have many questions: Do I need to take supplements for good health? If so, which ones do I need? How much is too much? Do supplements contain what they say they do? Who and what should I believe?

The National Academy of Sciences is updating its recommendations on vitamins and minerals. You may hear about Dietary Reference Intakes (DRIs), Recommended Dietary Allowances (RDAs) and the Tolerable Upper Intake Level (UL). Now experts are looking at what levels of vitamins and minerals are necessary to both prevent disease and promote good health, and how much is too much. RDAs are the dietary intakes that meet the nutritional requirements of nearly all individuals, and the UL is the maximum safe level of daily intake.

The following tables will help you get a better understanding of vitamins and minerals—what they do, how much is recommended (RDAs), common doses in supplements, Tolerable Upper Intake Level (UL) when available and, most importantly, the best food sources. The tables reflect dosages for healthy adults ages 18 and older.

Please note: First Place advises that you discuss the issue of vitamin and mineral supplementation with your personal physician. The following charts are for informational purposes only.

VITAMINS

There are 13 vitamins—four fat-soluble (A, D, E and K) and 9 water-soluble (C and the B vitamins). Compared to the major nutrients—carbohydrates, fats, proteins, and water—vitamins are only needed in small amounts, and they are not a source of energy for the body.

	ROLES AND FACTS	COMMON DOSAGES	GOOD SOURCES
Vitamin A	Maintains healthy cells, skin, and bones; important for vision and immune function. High doses can damage the liver. It's easy to get all the vitamin A you need from a healthy diet.	Women: 700 mcg[1]; Men: 900 mcg **UL is 3,000 mcg.**	Dairy products (cheese, butter, egg yolks); liver; fish oil; fortified foods; and dark green, yellow and orange vegetables.
Beta-carotene (Carotenoids)	Beta-carotene from plant sources is converted to vitamin A. Beta-carotene is an antioxidant that may protect the body from heart disease, cancer and cataracts.	No RDA— Supplements range from 2,500 to 25,000 IU[2] (1.5-15 mg[3]).	Look for fruits and vegetables with orange, red, yellow or dark green color (carrots, sweet potatoes, spinach, red bell pepper, apricots, mangoes and cantaloupe).

	ROLES AND FACTS	COMMON DOSAGES	GOOD SOURCES
Vitamin C	Antioxidant that protects your body's cells. Important for healthy skin, connective tissue, bone, and immune function. Large doses increase the risk of kidney stones.	60 mg— Supplements range from 60-500 mg. Women: 75 mg; Men: 90 mg. **UL is 2,000 mg.**	All citrus fruits, cantaloupe, strawberries, tomatoes, red and green bell peppers, potatoes and broccoli.
Vitamin D	Helps your body absorb calcium and phosphorous and build healthy bones. Too much vitamin D can cause kidney damage and weaken bones.	5 to 15 mcg (200-600 IU)— Supplements range from 100- 800 IU. **UL is 50 mcg (2,000 IU).**	Vitamin D is formed by the action of sunlight on the skin. Most milk products are fortified. Eggs, fish, margarine and fortified cereals also contain vitamin D.
Vitamin E	An antioxidant that protects your body's cells. It may protect against heart disease and cancer. It's been *claimed* to cure almost anything and slow the aging process.	Supplements range from RDA to 400 IU. 15 mg (22 in natural source, 33 in synthetic source). **UL is 1,000 mg** (1,500 in natural source, 1,100 in synthetic.)	Vegetable oils, nuts, seeds, salad dressings, margarine, wheat germ and green leafy vegetables.

	ROLES AND FACTS	COMMON DOSAGES	GOOD SOURCES
Vitamin K	Important for blood clotting; a deficiency of vitamin K is very unlikely because your body produces it from bacteria in the intestines and it's abundant in food.	Women: 65 mcg; Men: 80 mcg—No need to supplement.	Green leafy vegetables such as spinach and broccoli, peas, eggs, meat, milk, cereal and fruits.
Thiamin (Vitamin B1)	Important for energy production, metabolism and building healthy cells: proteins, blood and nerves.	Women: 1.1 mg; Men: 1.2 mg—Appears to be non-toxic.	Whole grains, fortified cereals, enriched grains, nuts, seeds and meats.
Riboflavin (Vitamin B2)	Important for energy production, metabolism and building healthy cells: proteins, blood and nerves.	Women: 1.1 mg; Men: 1.3 mg—Appears to be non-toxic.	Whole grains, fortified cereals, enriched grains, nuts, seeds, meats, dairy products and green leafy vegetables.
Niacin	Important for energy production, metabolism and building healthy cells: proteins, blood and nerves.	Women: 14 mg; Men: 16 mg—**UL is 35 mg.**	Same as riboflavin—meats are the best source.

	ROLES AND FACTS	COMMON DOSAGES	GOOD SOURCES
Vitamin B6 (Pyridoxine)	Important for energy production, metabolism and building healthy cells: proteins, blood and nerves. Reduces levels of homocysteine, which is associated with heart attack and stroke. High doses can cause nerve damage.	Women: 1.3-1.5 mg; Men: 1.3-1.7 mg—Supplements range from RDA to 50 mg. **UL is 100 mg.**	
Folate	Important for energy production, metabolism and building healthy cells: proteins, blood and nerves. Very important in pregnancy; reduces levels of homocysteine which is associated with heart attack and stroke.	400 mcg—**UL for supplementation is 1,000 mcg.**	Same as riboflavin; legumes and fortified cereals are important sources.
Vitamin B12	Important for energy production, metabolism and building healthy cells: proteins, blood and nerves. Reduces levels of homocysteine which is associated with heart attack and stroke.	2.4 mcg—Appears to be non-toxic.	Animal and fortified foods only.

	ROLES AND FACTS	COMMON DOSAGES	GOOD SOURCES
Biotin		30 mcg— Supplements range from 30 to 100 mcg.	Found in a wide variety of foods.
Panto-thenic Acid		5 mg—Appears to be nontoxic.	Found in a wide variety of foods.

Notes   1. mcg = micrograms   2. IU = international units   3. mg = milligrams

MINERALS

Just like vitamins, minerals play many important roles in the body.

	ROLES AND FACTS	COMMON DOSAGES	GOOD SOURCES
Calcium	Necessary for healthy bones. Plays an important role in muscle and nerve function and blood clotting. Low calcium intake increases the risk for osteoporosis. High calcium intake can cause kidney stones.	1,000-1,200 mg— Aim for 1,200 mg. Supplements range from 250 to 1,500 mg. UL is 2,500 mg.	Milk and dairy products (yogurt and cheese); dark green leafy vegetables; fortified foods such as juice, some cereals—tofu and soy milk are also good sources.
Chloride	Helps regulate fluid balance; important in digestion and nerve function.	No RDA—No need to supplement.	Salt.
Chromium	Works with insulin to regulate blood sugar. Studies don't support its role in promoting weight loss.	No RDA— Supplements range from 50 to 200 mcg.	Meat, eggs, whole grains and cheese.

	Roles and Facts	Common Dosages	Good Sources
Copper	Important in red blood cell formation and is a part of many enzymes.	90 mcg— Supplements range from 1-3 mg. **UL is 10,000 mcg.**	Seafood, nuts and seeds.
Flouride	Important for healthy bones and teeth.	Women: 3.1 mg; Men: 3.8 mg— Supplements range from 1.5 to 4 mg. **UL is 10 mg.**	Fluoridated drinking water and seafood.
Iodine	An important part of thyroid hormone which regulates metabolism.	150 mcg—Intakes of up to 2-3 mg appear safe.	Salt, seafood and some vegetables.
Iron	Needed to carry oxygen in the blood; avoid taking supplements with high doses of iron, unless prescribed by doctor.	Women:8-18 mg; Men:8 mg. **UL is 45 mg.**	Meats (the redder and darker the meat, the higher the iron), fortified cereals and grains, beans, nuts, seeds and dried fruits.
Magnesium	Important for healthy bones, nerves and muscles; a component of many enzymes.	Women: 320 mg; Men: 420 mg—**UL for supplementation is 350 mg.**	Legumes, nuts, whole grains and leafy green vegetables.

	ROLES AND FACTS	COMMON DOSAGES	GOOD SOURCES
Manga-nese	Component of many enzymes.	No RDA—supplements range from 2 to 5 mg. **UL is 11 mg.**	Whole grains, fruits and vegetables and tea.
Molyb-denum	Component of many enzymes.	45 mcg—supplements range from 75 to 250 mcg. UL **is 2,000 mcg.**	Milk, legumes and whole grains.
Phospho-rus	Important for healthy bones and teeth—helps regulate energy and maintain healthy cells.	700 mg: **UL is 3,000 to 4,000 mg.**	Dairy products, meats, legumes, nuts and eggs.
Potassium	Helps regulate fluid balance; important in muscle and nerve function.	No RDA— Supplements may contain 2,000 mg.	Fruits, vegetables and meats.
Selenium	Antioxidant that protects body's cells. May be protective against some cancers.	55 mcg—**UL is 400 mcg.**	Seafood, meats and eggs; grains, nuts and seeds.
Sodium	Helps regulate fluid balance; important in muscle and nerve function. A diet high in sodium may promote high blood pressure.	No RDA—No need to supplement. Limit to 2,400 mg/day.	

	Roles and Facts	Common Dosages	Good Sources
Zinc	Important for cell growth, immune function, wound healing and energy metabolism.	Women: 8 mg; Men: 11 mg. **UL is 40 mg.**	Meat, seafood, whole grains, nuts, seeds, milk and eggs.

summary and notes

It's important to try to meet your body's need for vitamins and minerals by following a healthy eating plan. If you decide that taking a supplement is right for you, try to stay within the dosages listed in these tables. Talk to your doctor about your personal needs.

The dosages listed in these charts may not be appropriate for children and adolescents.

If you're pregnant, breast-feeding your child or thinking about becoming pregnant, discuss your nutritional needs with your personal physician. The common dosages listed may not be appropriate if you're pregnant or breast-feeding your child.

The above common dosages may not apply to elderly individuals or people with underlying health problems. If you think you may have special nutritional needs, talk with your personal physician before taking any vitamin or mineral supplements.

understanding the nutrition facts panel

You don't need a degree in nutrition or chemistry to eat healthy. The Nutrition Facts Panel (NFP) gives you all you need to know. Learning to read labels can help you choose the foods that best fit into your healthy eating plan. The NFP provides information on calories, fat, saturated fat, cholesterol, fiber and other important nutrients in a single serving. The ingredients list tells you what's in a food, with ingredients listed from most to least. Food labels can also include nutrition and health claims.

Serving Size
The serving size is based on a typical portion, not necessarily the recommended serving. How does the serving size compare to what you eat? Controlling serving size is a great way to control your calorie intake.

Percent Daily Value
The Percent Daily Value, or % Daily Value, shows how one serving counts toward the recommended daily intake for specific nutrients. The percentage is based on a 2,000-calorie diet. Use the Percent Daily Value to see if a food is high or low in specific nutrients.

Calories
Keeping track of your daily calorie intake is a helpful strategy for losing weight. Use the NFP to help you monitor your eating habits. Calories from fat are indicated by the *number* of calories from fat, *not* the percentage. If you want to determine the percentage, divide the calories from fat by the total calories. On average, choose more foods with 30 percent or less of the calories from fat. Not every food you eat has to be less than 30 percent fat—just the overall balance of foods you eat!

Nutrients
Total fat, saturated fat, cholesterol, sodium, carbohydrates, fiber, sugars, protein, vitamins A and C, calcium and iron must be listed on the label. Vitamins and minerals added to foods must also be listed.

For total fat, saturated fat, cholesterol and sodium, look for foods with a low percent daily value.

For vitamins, minerals and fiber, your goal is to reach 100 percent each day. Choose foods with a high percentage of nutrients; a good source contains 10 percent or more.

At the bottom of the panel is the recommended amount of important nutrients for a 2,000 and a 2,500 calorie diet. It shows the maximum amounts of total fat, saturated fat, cholesterol and sodium recommended for a healthy and balanced eating plan: no more than 30 percent calories from fat, less than 10 percent saturated fat and less than 60 percent of total calories from carbohydrates. The last item on the panel is the number of calories per gram of fat, carbohydrate and protein.

A note about sodium: Although there is currently no Recommended Daily Intake (RDI)[1] for sodium, it is an electrolyte that is necessary for good health. Experts estimate that the body needs about 500 milligrams per day to maintain fluid balance, help muscles contract, aid in nerve transmissions and even regulate blood pressure. Most guidelines recommend that daily sodium consumption be limited to 2,400 or fewer milligrams—approximately 1 teaspoon of table salt, per day.[2] This amount is far less than the 4,000 to 6,000 milligrams consumed by the average American.

Understanding Nutrition and Health Claims

When it comes to health and nutrition claims, you can believe what you read. Food makers must meet strict government guidelines to list terms such as "low fat" or "reduced sodium" or to make health claims about heart disease, cancer or other diseases. Only health claims that are supported by scientific evidence and approved by the Food and Drug Administration (FDA) are allowed.

Understanding Terms

Calorie free	5 calories or fewer per serving
Low calorie	40 or fewer calories per serving
Fat free	Less than ½ (0.5) gram of total fat per serving
Low fat	3 or fewer grams of total fat per serving
Saturated fat free	Less than ½ (0.5) gram of saturated fat per serving
Low saturated fat	Less than 1 gram of saturated fat per serving
Cholesterol free	2 or fewer milligrams of cholesterol and 2 or fewer grams of saturated fat per serving
Low cholesterol	20 or fewer milligrams of cholesterol and 2 or fewer grams of saturated fat per serving
Sodium free	5 or fewer milligrams of sodium per serving
Low sodium	140 or fewer milligrams of sodium per serving
Very low sodium	35 or fewer milligrams of sodium per serving
Sugar free	Less than ½ (0.5) gram of sugar per serving
No sugar added	No sugars added during processing or packaging
Light or lite	⅓ less calories or 50 percent less of a nutrient such as fat, sodium or sugar than the regular or reference food
Reduced	25 percent less calories, fat, saturated fat, cholesterol, sodium or sugar than the regular or reference food; words such as "lower" and "fewer" might also be used
Lean	10 or fewer grams of fat, 4.5 or fewer grams of saturated fat and 95 or fewer milligrams of cholesterol per serving
Extra lean	5 or fewer grams of fat, 2 or fewer grams of saturated fat and 95 or fewer milligrams of cholesterol per serving

High	20 percent or more of the Percent Daily Value for a nutrient such as a vitamin, mineral or fiber; "excellent source of" and "rich in" may also be used
Good source	10 to 19 percent of the Percent Daily Value for a nutrient
More	10 percent or more of the Percent Daily Value for a nutrient; "enriched," "fortified" and "added" can also be used
Healthy	Low in fat and saturated fat, 480 or fewer milligrams of sodium and at least 10 percent of the Percent Daily Value of vitamin A, vitamin C, calcium, iron, protein and fiber per serving

Notes

1. "Reference Daily Intake" (RDI) is a new term that replaces "U.S. Recommended Daily Allowance" (RDA). The percentages that a food contributes to the RDI for these nutrients are listed on the food label.

2. One teaspoon of table salt is approximately 6,000 milligrams; however, table salt is made up of 40 percent sodium and 60 percent chloride.

what's the big deal about water?

You've probably heard more than once that you should drink eight 8-ounce glasses of water each day. Why the fuss? For starters, water makes up about 80 percent of your muscle mass, 60 percent of your red blood cells and more than 90 percent of your blood plasma. If you were stranded on a deserted island, you could go for weeks without food but only a few days without water. Take a look at the important role water plays in your body.

- It aids in the digestion and absorption of foods and nutrients.
- Water helps regulate the chemical reactions in every cell of your body.

- It transports nutrients and oxygen.
- Water is the vehicle your body uses to flush out the waste produced in normal body functions.
- It helps you maintain normal body temperature.
- Water is necessary for proper bowel function.
- It is responsible for maintaining proper fluid balance.

In your quest for healthy living, drinking plenty of water should be a top priority. In fact, if you're currently not drinking enough water, doing so will be one of the most significant lifestyle changes you can make.

Why Choose Water?

All fluids and some foods count toward your daily total of water. So why choose water? Water is good for you, it contains no calories, it's low in sodium, and it contains no additives or stimulants. Substituting water for calorie-containing beverages is an important step in helping you achieve and maintain a healthy body weight. Nonfat milk and 100 percent fruit juices are also good choices—they're packed with vitamins and minerals. However, watch the calories. The caffeine in tea, soft drinks and coffee acts as a stimulant and a diuretic (i.e., causes your body to lose water); thus, caffeine is not always a good choice. Choose God's abundant water as your number-one beverage!

Your body loses about 8 to 12 ounces of water throughout the day. To stay healthy and feel your best, you need to replace what your body loses. There's nothing magical about eight glasses of water a day; some people need a little more, some a little less. Drinking water throughout the day helps keep you ahead of the game.

Tap or Bottled?

Americans drink about 3.4 billion gallons of bottled water each year, and the numbers have been increasing about 10 percent per year. If drinking water from a bottle will encourage you to drink more, then bottled water is a good choice. However, don't assume that it's purer than tap water. In fact, according to the Natural Resources Defense Council (NRDC), some bottled waters may not be any better than tap water; they may even *be* tap water! In a recent study, the group found that one-third of 103 tested brands contained bacteria or other chemicals that exceed the industry's own guidelines or state purity standards.

While bottled water is safe, the NRDC noted that bottled-water companies tout the health benefits of their products and that consumers should be getting their money's worth. Since the study was released, legislation has been proposed for stricter standards on bottled water. Tap water is regulated under provisions of the Safe Drinking Water Act of 1974.

Eight Glasses a Day? That's Impossible!

Once you start drinking more water, your natural thirst for it will increase. With each glass you drink, think about the physical benefits. From time to time, review the list above that details how important water is to your body.

To make drinking water a habit, start by filling an eight-ounce measuring cup with water. Eight ounces is probably not as much as you think. What size glass will you use for those eight ounces? Another tactic is to fill a two-quart (64-ounce) container with water each morning and by noon make sure you have only one quart left. You're halfway to your goal!

You can keep a two-quart pitcher of water on your desk or in your refrigerator for easy access to water. Additionally, keep a water bottle in your car, take it to meetings and be sure to have water available when you exercise.

Tantalizing Tips

- Fill a pitcher with water, and add several orange slices for a light, refreshing flavor.
- Always ask for water when dining out, and try adding lemon or lime slices.
- Choose sparkling waters.

Dehydration

During the summer, you require more water because your body loses water through perspiration. If you live in a dry climate, your perspiration may evaporate more quickly so you might not sense the need to drink water, even though your body is still losing fluids. Don't wait for perspiration to be your warning sign to consume more water. The dry air in winter also increases your body's need for water. Don't wait until you feel thirsty to drink water; stay ahead of your thirst.

In addition to thirst, early signs of dehydration include the following:

- Fatigue
- Loss of appetite
- Flushed skin

- Light-headedness and dizziness
- Muscle cramping
- Infrequent urination and urine that's dark yellow

Water and Physical Activity

During physical activity, pay close attention to your water intake. Make sure you drink at least eight ounces before activity, and every 15 to 20 minutes during activity. You may need more when it's hot outside. To find out how much water you need to replenish your exercise losses, weigh yourself before and after exercise—the difference is mainly water. Replace one pound of weight loss with 16 ounces of water.

While the number on the scale may look better, dehydration is not a healthy way to lose weight. Avoid using sweatsuits or rubberized clothing to increase sweating during exercise. This is a dangerous practice and the weight you lose is only water—not fat! Body fat is made up of only 25 percent water compared to muscle, which is almost 80 percent water. Dehydration robs your body of the water it needs.

Unless you are an endurance athlete training for more than an hour, drink water rather than sports drinks.

An Essential Nutrient

While water is not included on the Food Guide Pyramid, don't ignore its importance. Next to air, you need water most for survival. Keep well hydrated and your body will perform better than ever. And you'll feel great too!

PLANNING FOR GOOD NUTRITION

stocking the healthy kitchen

Deciding you want to eat more healthfully is easy. It's much more difficult to actually make it happen! This can be particularly challenging for meals prepared at home. How many times have your intentions been good, but there just wasn't anything good to fix for dinner? If healthy food choices aren't kept in the kitchen, then the battle is lost before it's begun.

It is essential that your kitchen shelves reflect the new food goals you have set for yourself. Does this mean purchasing all fat-free, sugar-free and no-taste foods? Of course not! It does mean keeping certain foods on hand to provide you with lots of healthful choices. There are several things to consider as you begin planning your healthy kitchen.

Foods You Will Really Eat
Don't purchase foods because you *think* you should eat them. Purchase foods you *know* you'll eat. If rice cakes don't really suit your taste buds, don't buy them. Low-fat animal crackers or graham crackers may be more to your liking, so keep those on hand instead. You'll have to experiment a little to find what healthy foods you like best.

Frequency of Use
This is particularly important for cooking oils, flours, snack items, meat and fresh fruits and vegetables. Some foods might be used in small amounts—such as olive oil—and will last a long time. Buying in smaller quantities allows for greater freshness and less waste. Some foods tend to dry out and become stale quickly. It is better to buy single-serving sizes and enjoy all of them than to eat a few and throw out the rest. Using canned and frozen fruits and vegetables are

great choices, especially if you find your fresh versions are always spoiling before you eat them. Freezing breads and flours is a good way to preserve their freshness.

Preparation Time

For most people, time is a big consideration when planning a meal. Having a refrigerator stocked full of fresh produce and lean meat looks great, but if there isn't time to cook, it usually just ends up in the trash. Anticipate having a few times when you won't have time to cook. Keep some low-fat convenience foods on hand so you're not caught unprepared. Cooking extra and freezing the left-overs in single servings is a great way to have your own fast food!

List Making

After seriously considering your needs and preferences, go ahead and make out a kitchen list. Start by making a list of what you *normally* buy—no special foods or changes. Review your list to see if there are some items that you're willing to make healthy substitutions for. For example, you may be willing to substitute nonfat milk for 2% milk. Maybe the fried tortilla chips could be traded for baked chips or pretzels. You should also make a list of new foods you're willing to try.

Basic Items to Keep on Hand

In the Refrigerator

Cheese	Reduced-fat or low-fat cheeses are your best choices. When you only have time for a quick meal, a slice of cheese and whole-grain bread is a healthy choice. Grated cheese allows you to use less for the same amount of flavor. Choose sharp flavors.
Eggs	Eggs are a great source of lean protein, as well as a common ingredient for most baking. Learn to cook with egg whites and leave the yolk behind. Egg substitutes are also fine.
Fruits and vegetables	Make a list of your favorites and stock up every time you go to the store. Buy only what you can eat in one week. Cut up your vegetables when you first get home from the store so they're ready to go. Juices are also a good choice when you're on the run.

In the Refrigerator (continued)

Lunch meats	Keep a low-fat variety such as turkey or chicken breast on hand. Be sure to purchase in quantities that you actually eat! Try to choose low-sodium versions.
Milk	Keep plenty of low-fat (1%) or nonfat milk on hand; it's a great source of calcium.
Salad dressing	Choose "light," "low-fat," "reduced-fat," "nonfat" or "low-calorie" varieties; you may have to experiment to find one or two favorites.
Salad in a bag	It's washed and ready to go! Use nonfat or low-fat dressing.

In the Freezer

Frozen entrées	Choose entrées with 200 to 300 calories, 10 or fewer grams of fat and 400 or fewer milligrams of sodium.
Frozen vegetables	Buy in bags instead of boxes; allows you to use only what you need. You can buy individual servings too.
Snacks	Choose low-calorie items such as fruit bars or sherbet.

In the Pantry

Breakfast foods	Low-fat toaster pastries or granola bars for those grab-and-go mornings.
Canned foods	Keep canned vegetables such as corn, green beans, canned tomatoes, etc. These are commonly used items in casseroles and soups. Look for low-sodium varieties.
Cereal	Keep plenty of low-fat cereal around. Good choices are shredded wheat, bran cereals and oatmeal.
Herbs and spices	Make sure you have lots of herbs and spices on hand. Don't be afraid to try new ones! Keep a list of your favorites; replace them after about one year.
Nonstick spray	Essential for low-fat cooking. Specialty stores sell spray bottles to make your own.

In the Pantry (continued)

Oils	Choose at least one monounsaturated oil—olive or canola—and one polyunsaturated oil: corn, safflower or sunflower. Purchase only the amount you'll use over a few months, so it doesn't go bad before you use it.
Pasta	Always have a package of pasta ready to use! Choose a prepared pasta sauce that's low in fat. Prepackaged pasta dishes can be high in fat and sodium.
Rice	Add rice to a variety of meals. You may want to have two or three varieties, such as wild rice, basmati and your favorite flavored rice, but watch out for sodium.
Snacks	Choose only healthy snack foods: popcorn, low-fat cookies, low-fat snack crackers, rice cakes, dried fruits, etc. You can't eat what's not in the house!

Of course, this is not an exhaustive list, but it should get you headed in the right direction. With time you will discover the items you need in your kitchen for healthy eating. The trick is to stock a kitchen that works best for you and provides a variety of healthy foods to choose from anytime.

supermarket guide— solutions for healthy shopping

Do you realize that some of the most important health decisions you make are in the supermarket? That's right, healthy nutrition begins in the aisles of your grocery store! How do you decide what to buy when you shop?

- Do you purchase certain foods out of habit?
- Do you buy foods for taste or convenience?
- Do you usually choose those brands that are most familiar to you?
- Do you look for what's on sale or use coupons to help you decide?
- Do you read nutrition labels and comparison shop to help you choose the healthiest foods?

- Are you overwhelmed by the thousands of choices in the aisles of your grocery store?

No matter how you answered these questions, you can use this helpful shopping guide and your nutrition knowledge to choose those foods that will help you reach your goals for a healthy weight and good overall health.

Before You Shop
The best way to buy those foods that fit into your eating plan is to *plan ahead*.

Plan for Several Days at a Time
- What dishes will you be preparing?
- What foods will you need for breakfast, lunch and dinner?
- Will you be eating out during the week?
- Planning ahead will eliminate the wasted time of having to make a second or third trip to the store.

Check Your Cupboards, Refrigerator and Freezer
- Take stock of what you have, so you can use these foods first in upcoming meals.
- As you look, begin making a list of things you need from the store.

Prepare a List
- Keep an ongoing list in a convenient place in your kitchen.
- Add foods, supplies and ingredients to your list as you think of them.
- Use coupons only for foods that fit into your eating plan.
- Before you go shopping, compare your grocery list with your meal plan to make sure you have listed all the things you need.

Before You Leave
- Eat before you shop; never go to the store on an empty stomach!
- Plan on shopping during off-hours: early in the morning, late in the evening and midweek. When it's less crowded, you'll be more relaxed and have more time to make healthy decisions.
- Lace up your walking shoes so you can pick up the pace as you shop—every bit of physical activity counts! Plan on parking a little further away from the store entrance.

At the Store

- Rely on your list to help you stick to your shopping plan.
- First, walk around the outside aisles of your store. That's where you'll find the fresh produce, dairy products, baked goods, fresh meats, poultry and fish. Save the inside aisles, which contain more processed foods, for last.
- When it comes to shopping, try not to bring home foods that don't fit into your eating plan.
- Use food labels to help you make the healthiest choices, and limit foods with the following terms in the ingredients list:

Beef fat	Coconut oil	Lard
Butter	Hardened shortening	Palm kernel oil
Chicken fat	Hydrogenated shortening	Palm oil

tools for a healthy kitchen

Food choices and cooking methods are changing rapidly. Most of the recent changes reflect the desire of Americans to improve their health through better nutrition. Is your kitchen ready for this new way of cooking? While eating healthy doesn't require you to invest a lot of money in your kitchen, it's important to have the right equipment to get the job done. By keeping a few simple appliances and utensils handy, you'll always be ready to cook healthy. Having the right tools saves time and allows you to focus on other important things in life.

Having the right appliances, pots and pans, cooking utensils and storage containers can help you when cooking the healthy way. Start by surveying your kitchen to see what you have on hand.

Baking dishes and pans	Do you have the variety of shapes and sizes you need?
Blender	A blender can be used to purée, grate, chop and blend. It's also great for making healthy smoothies—a frozen fruit and dairy drink.
Cheese grater	Grating cheese allows you to use less—for the same amount of flavor. You can also use it for vegetables.
Egg separator	The egg yolk contains the fat and cholesterol. You can use only the egg whites in several recipes without affecting taste or texture.
Food processor	This machine allows you to purée, grate, chop and blend foods quickly.
Freezer bags	A great way to store leftovers. Keeping lots of different sizes on hand allows you to store large or small portions. Freezing in individual serving sizes provides quick meals that need little reheating time.
Gravy separator	Allows you to separate, or remove, unwanted fat from liquids. A kitchen syringe (meat baster) can also do the trick.
Herb and spice rack	Make flavorful seasonings convenient to use and store.
Hot-air popcorn popper	Requires no butter or oil. Add your own low-fat, no-salt seasonings.
Indoor/outdoor grill	Grilling allows the fat to drip freely from the meat.
Kitchen scale	This item is especially important when trying to determine portion sizes for foods such as meats, fish, chicken or cheese.
Kitchen scissors	Probably the easiest and quickest way to trim visible fat. Use your kitchen scissors only for food!
Measuring cups/spoons	Make sure you have plenty, so you can work with both wet and dry ingredients. The only way to learn about portion sizes is to measure everything you eat.
Meat thermometer	Takes the guesswork out of cooking meats and improves food safety.

Microwave	You probably have a microwave, but do you know how to take full advantage of all it can do?
Nonstick pots and pans	Make sure you have an assortment of nonstick pots and pans.
Nonstick skillet	This allows you to cook without adding fat. It also makes for easier cleanup!
Pastry brush	Perfect for when you need to put a light coat of oil on foods before cooking.
Plastic containers	These are great for the refrigerator. Clear containers let you see what is in them, so you are less likely to forget about leftovers. Some containers can go in the freezer as well as the microwave.
Plastic cutting board	Make sure you have a clean and safe surface for cutting and chopping. Clean your cutting board after every use with hot soapy water.
Roasting/broiling pan	Great for cooking meat the low-fat way—allows you to leave the fat behind.
Sharp knives	A good set of knives is indispensable to healthy and safe food preparation. Keep your knives sharpened and stored in a safe place.
Slotted spoon	Allows you to leave the fat and liquid behind.
Steamer	Steaming is a great way to cook vegetables, rice, poultry and fish.
Strainer or colander	Use it to strain and rinse the sodium from canned meats, legumes and vegetables. Use it to thaw frozen fruits and vegetables under running water. A microwave-safe strainer can be used to cook meats and collect fat drippings underneath.
Wok	A wok is a fast and easy way to prepare vegetables and stir-fry recipes. Most woks come with a nonstick surface, which allows you to use less oil (or no oil).

If your budget is tight, many of these will make terrific gifts for birthdays and holidays. If you don't have what you need to cook at home, are you more likely to eat out? Investing in the right tools saves money in the long run.

Organizing Your Kitchen

Not only is it important to have the tools you need, it's important to be organized.

- Keep your kitchen counter space clean and clear of junk (e.g., mail, newspapers, magazines and whatever else might be lying around).
- Organize pots, pans and other cooking utensils for easy use and storage.
- Clean dishes as you cook, which saves time in the long run.
- Assemble all ingredients and utensils in one place. Make sure you have everything you need before you start to cook.

AN OUNCE OF PREVENTION

controlling cholesterol

Today, almost everyone knows something about cholesterol. In fact, many people even know their blood cholesterol numbers. However, with what seems like a new report on cholesterol every day, it's often hard to know what to do.

Believe it or not, cholesterol is important for good health. It's used to make certain hormones, it helps digest fat, and it's an essential part of every cell membrane. Your blood cholesterol levels are influenced by several factors: heredity, diet, physical activity, body weight and other lifestyle habits.

The foods you eat can have a big impact on your blood cholesterol level. Eating foods high in saturated fat and cholesterol can raise your cholesterol level. Too much cholesterol in the bloodstream increases the chances that your blood vessels will become blocked with fats, cholesterol and other components. This blockage can lead to heart attack and stroke.

Did You Know?
- Cholesterol is not a fat—it's a fatlike substance.
- Saturated fat actually raises blood cholesterol levels more than dietary cholesterol does.
- Cholesterol is not found in plant foods—fruits, vegetables or grains. Saturated fat, however, is found in some plant foods: palm oil, palm kernel oil and coconut oil.
- Your body makes all the cholesterol it needs; it's not necessary to get cholesterol from food.
- Children younger than two years of age should not follow a low-fat, low-cholesterol eating plan. Fat and cholesterol are necessary for normal growth and development and a healthy nervous system.

Understanding Cholesterol Levels

When most people talk about their cholesterol level, they're talking about total cholesterol. The higher your total cholesterol, the higher your risk for heart disease. However, there's more to blood cholesterol than the total cholesterol level alone. Cholesterol is carried in your body in special packages called lipoproteins.

The two most important lipoproteins are *LDL cholesterol* and *HDL cholesterol*. Think of the *L* in LDL as standing for *lousy*. This is the bad cholesterol that tends to block arteries. People who have too much LDL have a higher risk of heart disease. Think of the *H* in HDL as standing for *helpful*. HDL is the good cholesterol that carries cholesterol away from the arteries. People who have a high level of HDL have a lower risk of heart disease.

You may also have heard about *triglycerides*. In your body, fat is carried in the bloodstream in the form of triglycerides. Triglycerides and cholesterol are often carried together in the same packages. High blood triglycerides levels appear to be associated with an increased risk of heart disease in some people.

Know Your Numbers

Do your cholesterol levels meet these recommended levels?

Total cholesterol less than 200 mg/dL	☐ Yes	☐ No
LDL cholesterol less than 130 mg/dL	☐ Yes	☐ No
HDL cholesterol higher than 40 mg/dL	☐ Yes	☐ No
Triglycerides less than 200 mg/dL	☐ Yes	☐ No

Did you answer no to any of these? If so, you may have abnormal cholesterol levels. If you have abnormal blood cholesterol levels—particularly high LDL cholesterol—experts agree that lowering your blood cholesterol can reduce your risk of having a heart attack. Recent studies show that lowering your cholesterol level can prevent certain types of strokes, too. Talk to your doctor about what's best for you. If you don't know your numbers or you haven't had your cholesterol checked in several years, make an appointment with your doctor for a checkup.

Your Low-Cholesterol Lifestyle

Everyone needs to follow an eating plan that's low in fat, saturated fat and cholesterol and high in whole grains, fruits and vegetables. It is also important to achieve and maintain a healthy body weight—losing weight lowers cholesterol levels. Physical activity is important because it raises the good HDL cholesterol and helps you maintain a healthy weight. Smoking lowers HDL levels.

Choose	Instead of
Lean meats, poultry and fish with visible fat and skin removed.	Fatty cuts of meat, organ meats (liver, kidneys) or other high-fat meats (sausage, bacon).
3 to 6 ounces of meat each day— 3 ounces is about the size of an audiocassette.	Typical restaurant-sized portions of 8 to 12 ounces.
Fat-free or low-fat milk or yogurt, and some low-fat cheese.	2% or whole milk or full-fat yogurt, cheese or cheese spreads.
Margarine that lists liquid vegetable oil or water as the first ingredient.	Butter or margarine that lists hydrogenated vegetable oil as the first ingredient.
Vegetable oils (canola, olive, saf-flower, corn) and low-fat salad dressings or mayonnaise.	Shortening, tropical oils (palm and coconut), mayonnaise or full-fat dressings.
Low-fat cooking methods: broil, bake, grill, roast or poach.	Frying or cooking with heavy creams, cheese and sauces.
More fruits, vegetables and whole grains every day.	Meat and highly processed breads, cereals and snack foods.

Counting Cholesterol and Saturated Fat

Use this table to compare the cholesterol, saturated fat and total fat in various foods.

	Total Fat (g)	Saturated Fat (g)	Cholesterol (mg)
Liver (3 ounces, cooked)	4	2	333
Eggs (1 whole)	5	2	213
*Shrimp (8 medium)	2	1	167
Hamburger (3 ounces, cooked)	17	8	77
Lean beef (3 ounces, cooked)	8	3	72
Baked, skinless chicken breast (3 ounces, cooked)	3	1	72
Whole milk (1 cup)	8	5	33
Natural cheddar cheese (1 ounce)	9	6	29
Glazed doughnut (1 medium)	10	2	18
Skim milk (1 cup)	1	trace	4
Whole wheat bread (1 slice)	1	trace	0
Fruits and vegetables, except avocados and olives	trace	trace	0

* Shellfish, such as shrimp, were once considered off-limits because of their high cholesterol content. However, because they're low in saturated fat, they can be a heart-healthy choice—but not if battered and fried!

preventing cancer

Scientific evidence suggests that nearly 30 percent of cancer deaths are related to dietary factors. In fact, experts predict that for the majority of Americans who don't smoke, dietary and physical activity habits are the most important modifiable risk factors for cancer. There is little doubt that nutrition plays a role in contributing to and preventing cancer. A definitive answer about the optimal diet for preventing cancer and which nutrients have specific effects is not yet known.

What Is Cancer?

Cancer is a group of diseases caused by the abnormal growth and spread of the body's cells. When these cells grow out of control, they can develop into cancerous (malignant) tumors. Cancers result in death by interfering with several of the body's normal processes.

Many factors contribute to cancer, including heredity, aging, environment and lifestyle. For example, a smoker's risk of developing lung cancer is 10 times higher than that of a nonsmoker. A woman with a mother, sister or daughter with breast cancer has twice the risk of developing breast cancer as a woman who does not have such a family history. Too much exposure to the sun's rays increases the risk for skin cancer. Early detection and eliminating risk factors are very important aspects of preventing cancer and cancer deaths.

Cancer and Nutritional Health

Several groups publish nutrition guidelines to advise the public about dietary practices that reduce risk of cancer. Current recommendations are based on the consensus of hundreds of experts and thousands of scientific studies. The following are consistent with dietary recommendations from the American Cancer Society, National Cancer Institute, World Cancer Research Fund and the American Institute for Cancer Research:

- **Choose most of the foods you eat from plant sources.** Eat five or more servings of fruits and vegetables each day. Especially try to choose dark green and yellow vegetables, vegetables in the cabbage family, soy products and legumes.

    Eat 6 to 11 servings a day of grains including breads, cereals, rice and pasta. Choose mostly whole grains instead of highly processed or refined grains.

- **Limit your intake of high-fat foods, particularly those from animal sources.** Select lean cuts and smaller portions when you eat meat, use low-fat cooking techniques, select nonfat or low-fat dairy products and replace high-fat foods with fruits, vegetables, grains and legumes.
- **Get 30 minutes or more of moderate-intensity activity on most days each week.**
- **Achieve and maintain a healthy weight.**
- **Limit consumption of alcoholic beverages—if you drink at all.**

Scientific Evidence

- Fruits and vegetables contain over 100 beneficial vitamins, minerals, fiber and phytochemicals (plant chemicals), many of which may protect against cancer. Some of the nutrients that may be specifically beneficial include the antioxidant vitamins, fiber, calcium, folate, selenium, carotenoids, flavinoids and sulfurophanes. Studies show that an increased consumption of fruits and vegetables reduces the risk of certain types of cancer. The evidence is particularly strong for colon cancer.
- High-fat diets, particularly saturated fats, are associated with an increase in the risk of cancers of the colon and rectum, prostate and endometrium (uterus).
- Consumption of meat, particularly red meat, has been associated with certain cancers. What's the best advice? Limit meat intake to the recommended servings and portion sizes (3 to 6 ounces); choose lean cuts of meat, poultry (without the skin), fish and meat alternatives such as legumes instead of high-fat red meats; and avoid charring meat over a direct flame.
- Physical activity may help protect against cancer of the colon, breast, prostate and endometrium. The protective effects may be related to energy balance and hormone levels.
- Obesity also appears to increase the risk of developing certain cancers.
- Alcoholic beverages are associated with an increased risk of cancer in the oral cavity, esophagus, larynx and breast.

Cancer Screening

Cancer screening is one of the most important steps you can take to increase your chances of surviving cancer. Regular screening examinations are currently recommended for the breast, cervix, colon, oral cavity, prostate, rectum, testes and skin. Self-examinations of the breast, testes and skin are important steps in detecting cancer early. A regular medical checkup can also detect cancers of the thyroid, lymph nodes, ovaries and other areas of the body. Here is a cancer-related checkup schedule recommended by the American Cancer Society.

Breast

Monthly self-examination should begin at age 20, with clinical examinations every three years for women aged 20 to 40; then yearly after age 40.

The American Cancer Society recommends yearly mammograms beginning at age 40, although some groups recommend at least one mammogram between the ages of 40 and 50 and then yearly mammograms beginning at age 50. Talk to your doctor about what is best for you.

Cervical

Beginning at age 18 (or with the initiation of sexual activity), young women should have a yearly Pap test and pelvic examination.

Colon and Rectum

Regular screening of the colon and rectum should begin at age 50 (if you have a strong family history of colon cancer or polyps, you may need to begin screening earlier). Tests usually involve a yearly examination for blood in the stool and a rectal examination.

Every 5 to 10 years one of the following tests to look at the inside of the colon should also be performed: a sigmoidoscopy, a colonoscopy or a barium enema. Talk to your doctor about the screening test and schedule that is best for you.

Prostate

Beginning at age 50, men should have yearly digital rectal examinations and Prostate-Specific Antigens (PSA).

African-Americans and men with a strong family history of cancer may want to begin screening earlier. Talk to your doctor about what's best for you.

preventing diabetes

Diabetes is a serious disease and is the seventh leading cause of death in the United States. Sixteen million Americans have diabetes, and one in three don't even know they have it! Each year, nearly 800,000 people are diagnosed and over 190,000 deaths result from diabetes. Diabetes kills more women each year than breast cancer. Diabetes is very damaging to the body and is a major cause of blindness, kidney disease, nerve damage and amputations. People with diabetes have two to four times the risk of heart attack and stroke.

Types of Diabetes

Diabetes means that your blood sugar—glucose—is too high. Your blood always has some sugar in it because your body requires a constant supply of sugar for energy. However, too much sugar in the blood is not good for your health. Most of the food you eat is converted into glucose—sugar—for energy. For the glucose to get into the body's cells a hormone called insulin must be present. In a person who has diabetes, either the body does not produce enough insulin or the cells don't use it properly. As a result, blood-sugar levels rise. There are two major types of diabetes.

Type 1 Diabetes

Type 1 Diabetes is an autoimmune disease in which the body does not produce enough insulin. It usually begins in childhood or young adulthood. Without enough insulin, the body cannot control blood sugar. The only way to survive with type 1 diabetes is to take daily injections of insulin. Type 1 accounts for only 5 to 10 percent of all diabetes sufferers.

Type 2 Diabetes

Type 2 Diabetes results from an inability to make enough insulin or properly use it—insulin resistance. Type 2 is the most common form of diabetes and accounts for 90 to 95 percent of cases. This form of diabetes usually develops in adults over the age of 45. Nearly 80 percent of people with type 2 diabetes are overweight. Type 2 diabetes is on the rise due to the increasing age, weight and sedentary lifestyles of Americans.

Risk Factors for Type 2 Diabetes—Doctors don't yet understand all the reasons people develop type 2 diabetes. The following factors (many of which can be lowered with healthy lifestyle habits) are associated with a higher risk:

- Family history of type 2 diabetes in a parent or sibling
- Overweight and obesity
- A sedentary lifestyle
- A history of diabetes during pregnancy or delivery of a baby weighing more than nine pounds
- Low HDL cholesterol ($\leq$ 40 mg/dL) or high trigycerides ($\geq$ 200 mg/dL)
- High blood pressure ($\geq$ 140/90)
- African-Americans, Hispanics and Native Americans have a higher risk

Diagnosis

Experts now recommend that adults 45 years and older be tested for diabetes. If you're under 45 years of age and you have one or more risk factors for diabetes, you should also be tested. Early diagnosis and treatment can lower the risk of the serious complications associated with diabetes. The best way to test for diabetes is to have a blood test performed after you haven't eaten anything for at least eight hours. This is called a fasting plasma glucose test. Do you know your blood sugar level?

Risk Classification	Fasting Plasma Glucose Level	My Level
Normal	< 110 mg/dL	
Increased Risk	110 to 125 mg/dL	
Diabetes	$\geq$ 126 mg/dL	

If your blood glucose is normal, take lifestyle steps to keep it that way and have repeat testing every three years. If your level puts you at an increased risk, ask your doctor about further testing. If you have diabetes, you need to take your blood sugar levels very seriously. If you have diabetes, you need to work with your doctor and a registered dietitian to do all you can to keep your blood sugar under control.

Prevention

There are several things you can do to lower your risk for type 2 diabetes. If you're at risk, it's important that you do all you can to prevent diabetes. Fortunately, following a healthy lifestyle will help you keep your risk low. In addition to living a healthy lifestyle, make sure to get regular medical checkups.

- **Follow a healthy eating plan.** Healthy eating can help to keep your risk low. The most important thing is to maintain a healthy body weight. A healthy eating plan is high in fruits, vegetables and whole grains, and low in foods that are high in fat, saturated fat and cholesterol.
- **Control your weight.** Weight gain is associated with increasing risk for diabetes—the higher your weight, the higher your risk. If you're overweight, a weight loss of as little as 5 to 10 percent can significantly reduce your chances of developing diabetes.
- **Exercise regularly.** A sedentary lifestyle and low level of physical fitness is associated with an increased risk for developing diabetes. Regular physical activity and exercise help your body use insulin and sugar more efficiently. Physical activity also helps you achieve and maintain a healthy weight and lowers your risk for heart disease. Are you fitting in at least 30 minutes of physical activity several days each week?

preventing heart disease

Diseases of the heart and blood vessels—cardiovascular disease—claim nearly 1 million lives in the United States each year. That's one death every three seconds! Coronary heart disease (CHD), which causes heart attacks, is the leading killer of both men and women. Each year over 1 million heart attacks occur and nearly 500,000 result in death—one-half of these victims are women! Stroke, another form of cardiovascular disease, is the third leading killer of men and women.

The Causes of Heart Attacks and Strokes

Arteriosclerosis is the underlying process that causes most heart disease. It results from the buildup of fat, cholesterol and cells in the lining of the arteries. This buildup is called plaque and as it progresses, the flow of blood to the heart or brain can be blocked, or the plaque can rupture, causing a heart attack or stroke. While a heart attack or a stroke can occur suddenly, arteriosclerosis develops as a result of many years of unhealthy choices.

The Eight Major Risk Factors

There are now eight major risk factors for heart disease. The more factors a person has, the greater the risk of heart attack and stroke. Notice that the first two are factors that cannot be changed, but the rest can be avoided by making lifestyle changes.

1. **Age**—Men aged 45 or older and women 55 and older are at a higher risk. The risk for women seems to increase most dramatically after menopause.

   What is your age? _____

2. **Family History**—Your risk is higher if you have a family history of heart disease—a male relative who had a heart attack before the age of 55 or female relative before the age of 65.

   Do you have a family history of coronary disease? ☐ Yes ☐ No

3. **Smoking**—A smoker's risk of heart attack is twice that of a nonsmoker. Secondhand smoke also increases your risk. A smoker is much more likely to die when a heart attack or stroke occurs than a nonsmoker. If you smoke, make every possible effort to quit.

   Are you currently a smoker? ☐ Yes ☐ No

4. **Abnormal Cholesterol Levels**—The risk of heart disease rises as the total and LDL cholesterol (the bad cholesterol) levels increase. The risk of heart disease also rises as HDL cholesterol (the good cholesterol) levels decrease. High triglycerides may also increase your risk.

What are your cholesterol levels? Write your levels in the appropriate boxes.

Risk	Low		Borderline		High	
	Range	My Score	Range	My Score	Range	My Score
Total Cholesterol	< 200		200-239		≥ 240	
LDL Cholesterol	< 130		130-159		≥ 160	
HDL Cholesterol	> 40				≤ 40	
Triglycerides	< 200				≥ 200	

If your numbers are in the high or borderline range and you have two or more other risk factors, you may be greatly adding to your risk of a heart attack or stroke. Talk to your doctor. Treatment and prevention always involve lifestyle changes such as following a diet low in saturated fat and cholesterol, achieving and maintaining a desirable weight and exercising regularly.

5. **High Blood Pressure**—High blood pressure increases the risk of heart attack and stroke. A blood pressure greater than 140/90 is high. Even pressures slightly lower—135-139/85-89—can put you at greater risk.

   What is your blood pressure? Write it in the appropriate box.

Risk	Low	Borderline	High
Scale	< 130/80	130-139/85-89	≥140/90
My Blood Pressure			

If your blood pressure is high, talk to your doctor. Treatment and prevention always involve lifestyle changes such as weight control, physical activity and restriction of alcohol and sodium intake. An eating plan high in fruits and vegetables (7 to 10 servings) and low-fat dairy products (2 to 3 servings) may also help lower blood pressure.

6. **Physical Inactivity**—A sedentary lifestyle increases the risk of heart disease nearly two times. This risk is as high as that caused by abnormal cholesterol levels, high blood pressure *and* cigarette smoking combined. Despite the known risks, 60 percent of adults and 30 percent of children don't get enough physical activity to benefit their health. Regular moderate physical activity cuts your risk of dying from heart disease in half.

Are you getting at least 30 minutes of moderate physical activity several days each week?　☐ Yes　☐ No

7. **Obesity and Overweight**—Excess body fat increases the risk for both heart attack and stroke. Obesity is also associated with increased blood pressure, abnormal cholesterol levels and diabetes. Losing just 10 percent of excess weight and keeping it off can significantly lower risk.

Are you within your healthy weight range?　☐ Yes　☐ No

8. **Diabetes**—Diabetes (high blood sugar) is very damaging to the heart and blood vessels. If you or a loved one has diabetes, it's important to do all you can to control blood sugar and other risk factors. A fasting blood sugar level greater than 125 mg/dL indicates diabetes.

What is your fasting blood sugar level? _____

preventing osteoporosis

Osteoporosis is one of the most significant health problems in this country. Over 25 million Americans, mostly postmenopausal women, are affected by osteoporosis—but men can be affected too. Osteoporosis results in over 1.5 million fractures each year. Unfortunately, in the elderly many of these fractures result in significant disability—even death! The seriousness of osteoporosis makes low calcium intake one of the most important nutrition-related problems in the country. Only 20 percent of women meet the daily recommended intake for calcium. A sedentary lifestyle is also a major risk factor.

What Is Osteoporosis?

Osteoporosis is a weakening of the bones that results from the gradual loss of calcium and other minerals. These weak bones can easily fracture during a fall. They can even break during normal activities. The spine, hip and wrist are the most common sites for fracture. Unfortunately, this disease is often silent and the first symptoms are fracture and disability.

Fortunately, osteoporosis can be prevented—and treated. Prevention is best begun in childhood because the amount of bone—what doctors call peak bone mass—achieved before the age of 35 is an important predictor of risk. The key to prevention is building healthy bones through good nutrition, regular physical activity, a healthy lifestyle and medical therapy when appropriate—it's never too late to start!

Risk Factors

Check off risk factors that may affect you.

☐ I am a Caucasian or Asian woman.

☐ I am underweight or small boned.

☐ There is a history of osteoporosis in my family.

☐ I am postmenopausal. (The rate of bone loss increases rapidly after menopause, whether natural or surgical. The body's estrogen helps women maintain and build healthy bones.)

Tips

• Hormone replacement therapy (HRT) can slow bone loss after menopause. Talk to your doctor to see if hormones are right for you.

• Regular weight-bearing physical activity throughout life builds healthy bones. How active are you?

• Smoking promotes bone loss. If you smoke, quit!

• Calcium and other vitamins and minerals are essential for good bone health. How's your calcium intake?

• Diets high in protein, sodium and caffeine have little effect on bone health. Unfortunately, soft drinks, tea and coffee often replace good sources of calcium, such as nonfat milk and fortified orange juice.

• Eating disorders such as bulimia and anorexia nervosa are associated with poor bone health and osteoporosis.

Calcium Needs

Calcium is essential for bone health, but it also has several other important roles in the body such as nerve function, muscle contraction and blood clotting. The body contains more calcium than any other mineral. Most of your calcium—99 percent—is stored in your bones. If you don't get enough calcium from your diet, your body steals it from your bones. Milk, yogurt and cheese supply

75 percent of dietary calcium. A high intake of dietary calcium may also prevent high blood pressure and colon cancer.

Although it's easy to get all the calcium you need from a healthy eating plan, the majority of women only get about half of the calcium they need for bone health. Most adults should get around 1,200 milligrams of calcium each day. If your risk for osteoporosis is high, some experts recommend 1,500 milligrams. Check out the following high-calcium eating plan:

Three servings of low-fat dairy (a serving is 8 ounces of milk or yogurt)	~ 900 to 1,000 mg
1 to 1.5 oz. of cheese (a single sandwich slice or a cube the size of your thumb)	~ 200 mg
8 ounces of calcium-fortified orange juice	~ 300 mg
Healthful diet (dark green leafy vegetables, fruits, whole grains and legumes)	~ 200 to 400 mg
Total	~ 1,600 to 1,900 mg

If you're lactose intolerant or a strict vegetarian (no dairy), it can be more difficult to meet your daily calcium needs. Many people who are lactose intolerant can drink smaller servings of milk—start with 2- to 4-ounce servings—or drink it with meals. Yogurt, cheese and buttermilk are often easier to digest. Try using a reduced lactose milk or lactase enzyme. Other good sources of calcium include tofu processed with calcium and calcium-fortified foods such as orange juice, soy milk and cereals. Make sure to eat lots of dark green leafy vegetables, fruits, whole grains, legumes and nuts, too.

What About Calcium Supplements?

Food sources are your first choice because they contain other important nutrients your body needs. However, if your diet falls short, a supplement may be a good idea. Talk to your doctor about what's best for you. If you choose to supplement, only supplement the amount of calcium you need—small doses of 250 to 500 milligrams are best. It's best to take a calcium supplement with a meal to help absorption. Calcium carbonate and calcium citrate are good sources. Daily intake of calcium greater than 2,500 milligrams increase the risk of kidney stones.

The Role of Physical Activity

Studies show that active men and women have healthier bones. The bones adapt to the stress of regular weight-bearing physical activity by becoming stronger. Good activities include walking, jogging, aerobics, strength training and recreational sports that keep you on your feet. Recent studies show that strength training can slow down and even reverse the loss of bone that occurs in postmenopausal women. Doing some activity in the sunshine a few days a week can give you an additional boost—more vitamin D!

A Word About Vitamin D

Vitamin D is also important—it helps your body use calcium to build healthy bones. If you drink milk, you're likely getting enough vitamin D. Your skin can also produce vitamin D with the help of sunshine; 10 to 15 minutes a few days each week is all you need. If you don't drink milk or you get little sunshine, you may need to consider a supplement.

understanding high blood pressure

Fifty million—nearly one out of four—Americans have high blood pressure. More than half of all Americans over the age of 65 have high blood pressure! Unfortunately, many people are not aware they have it. High blood pressure is often called the silent killer because it usually causes no symptoms. If your blood pressure is high, you're at a much greater risk for heart attack, stroke and kidney disease. It's important to know your blood pressure and take steps to bring it down if it's high. A healthy lifestyle can lower your risk of developing high blood pressure in the future.

What Is Blood Pressure?

You've probably had your blood pressure measured before, but you may not know what the two numbers mean. The numbers tell you how hard your blood is pressing on the walls of your arteries as it flows through your body. If your blood pressure is high, your heart and arteries are working too hard. High blood pressure can damage the heart, arteries and organs such as the brain and kidneys. The first or top number is the systolic pressure. This is the pressure created in the arteries when the heart contracts. The second or bottom number is the diastolic pressure. This is the pressure in the arteries when the heart relaxes between beats. What are your blood-pressure numbers?

Risk	Systolic (mmHg)	Diastolic (mmHg)	My Blood Pressure
Optimal	120	80	
Normal	120 to 129	80 to 84	
High Normal	130 to 139	85 to 89	
High	140	90	

If your blood pressure is 140/90 or greater, talk to your doctor and begin making healthful lifestyle changes today. If you're in the high normal range, watch your blood pressure very closely. If you don't know your blood pressure, get it measured. No matter what your blood pressure, a healthy lifestyle can help you keep it low.

Causes of High Blood Pressure
Doctors don't know all the factors that cause high blood pressure. In at least 90 percent of people the cause is unknown. In such cases, the diagnosis is called "primary" or "essential" hypertension. High blood pressure often runs in families and the risk increases with age. Several lifestyle factors also seem to be associated with high blood pressure: weight gain and obesity, a sedentary lifestyle and poor dietary habits.

Prevention of High Blood Pressure
Fortunately, a healthy lifestyle can lower your chances of developing high blood pressure or help lower it if it's already high. Doctors now recommend "the big five" lifestyle strategies to control blood pressure.

Achieve and Maintain a Healthy Weight
As your body weight rises, blood pressure often rises too. If you are overweight, losing as little as 10 percent of your weight can significantly decrease your risk of developing high blood pressure or lower it if it's high. Losing weight can also lower your risk for heart attack, stroke and diabetes. Monitor your blood pressure every few months as you lose weight.

Get and Stay Physically Active

Regular, moderate physical activity can lower your blood pressure and improve your health and well-being. Try to do at least 30 minutes of activity on most, preferably all, days of the week. Brisk walking, gardening, bicycling and swimming are good examples of moderate activities. Pick activities that you enjoy and make them a part of your everyday life. Select an activity that requires some exertion but is comfortable and enjoyable. Continue this activity on a regular basis; when it becomes less challenging, gradually increase the time or intensity or add another activity you enjoy. You don't have to do 30 minutes at one time. You can break it into sessions of 10 to 15 minutes two or three times a day. This may help you get started.

Follow a Healthy Eating Plan

For years, doctors have known the benefits of cutting down on sodium and alcohol intake. In fact, studies show that the combination of modest weight loss and limited sodium intake can reverse high blood pressure in many people. The latest news on controlling blood pressure, however, comes from a study called DASH—Dietary Approaches to Stop Hypertension. The DASH study found that eating the right foods can lower blood pressure as effectively as taking medication.

The DASH Diet

- High in fruits and vegetables—7 to 10 servings daily.
- High in low-fat dairy foods—2 to 3 servings daily.
- High in grains (breads, cereal, rice and pasta)—6 or more servings daily.
- Moderate amounts of lean meat, chicken or fish daily—no more than 2 servings daily.
- Legumes, nuts and seeds—4 to 5 servings weekly (more beans than nuts or seeds).
- Low in fat and saturated fat—no more than 2 to 3 daily servings of fats such as oils, margarine, mayonnaise or salad dressing.
- Low in sweets—no more than 5 low-fat sweets each week. Fruit is the preferred dessert.
- The DASH study did not involve efforts to lose weight or restrict sodium.

The DASH researchers don't understand all the reasons that this eating plan is so beneficial. One reason may be its high potassium, magnesium and calcium content.

There is good evidence that salt restriction can lower blood pressure. Higher salt intake is related to higher blood pressure in some people. Cutting back on salt and sodium may help keep blood pressure low. Use less salt in cooking and at the table. Most salt and sodium come from processed and fast foods. Learn to read labels and buy low-salt alternatives.

Reducing alcohol intake can also lower blood pressure. In addition to increasing blood pressure, excessive alcohol consumption can cause a variety of other serious health problems, such as liver, kidney or heart disease.

WHAT'S COOKING?

changing recipes

Low-fat cookbooks fill bookstore and library shelves. Perhaps you even have a collection of favorite cookbooks. If you like to cook and learn new recipes, that's great. But for most of us, learning all new recipes is not realistic. You don't have to buy a new cookbook or learn all new recipes to eat healthy and lose weight. You can make almost any recipe healthier with a few simple changes. Use the following tips to help turn your recipes into healthier alternatives.

Just for Starters
- Which ingredients can be changed? Start by looking at ways to cut calories, fat, sugar and sodium.
- Find ways to increase nutrition by adding or substituting more healthful foods, such as whole grains, vegetables, legumes and fruits for less healthful foods, such as high-fat meats and refined grains.
- Make changes gradually to learn what works best. Changing ingredients can affect taste, texture and appearance.
- For that special occasion, don't change your favorite recipe—serve smaller portions.

Cut the Fat
- Instead of frying meat, poultry and fish, broil, grill, roast or bake them. Use a rack or pans designed to catch drippings so that meat won't cook in its own fat. Use lean meats trimmed of visible fat and skin.
- Use vegetable-oil spray and nonstick pots and pans instead of oils and butter for cooking. Baste, broil and stir-fry using small amounts of oil, broth, water or fruit juice.

- Limit meat portions in your recipes to three ounces or less per serving. Make up for the reduced meat by adding more grains, rice or pasta, vegetables or legumes.
- Use meat alternatives—beans, lentils, peas and soy products—in recipes calling for meat.
- Drain fat from meat during or after cooking. Rinse cooked ground meat with hot water to remove much of the fat.
- Refrigerate soups and stews before serving. Remove the layer of fat that hardens after cooling.
- In recipes calling for eggs, use cholesterol-free egg substitutes or substitute two egg whites for every whole egg.
- To cut the fat called for in a recipe by ⅓ to ½, substitute vegetable oils instead of butter or shortening, and use low-fat dairy products.
- In recipes calling for cheese, use ⅓ to ½ of what the recipe calls for. Use low-fat cheese with 3 to 5 grams of fat per 1-ounce serving.
- Use nonfat sour cream or make your own by mixing ½ cup of low-fat yogurt and ½ cup of low-fat cottage cheese. Flavor with lemon juice and your favorite herbs and spices.
- Replace some of the fat in baked goods with fruit purées, such as prune, apple-sauce or banana, or nonfat dairy products such as nonfat yogurt. Use ½ cup of puréed fruit in place of 1 cup of butter, shortening or oil. Don't get rid of all the fat. You may need to add 1 to 2 tablespoons of fat back into the recipe to achieve the best results.
- Use low-fat or nonfat cream cheese, sour cream, yogurt, mayonnaise and salad dressing instead of the full-fat versions.

Cut the Sugar

- Try using ⅓ less sugar than what the recipe calls for.
- Substitute artificial sweeteners when appropriate. This will not work in many baked goods. Aspartame (e.g., NutraSweet, Equal) is not the best choice for cooking—it loses its sweetness at temperatures over 350°. Sucralose (e.g., Splenda), however, can be used in cooking and baking.
- Learn to make special treats with fruits, such as fruit and yogurt smoothies, fruit pops, frozen bananas and trail mix.
- Experiment using fruit juice concentrates instead of sugar. You'll need to reduce the amount of overall liquid ingredients.
- Serve smaller portions of your favorite recipes.

Cut the Sodium

- Add flavor to vegetables, meats, poultry and fish with herbs and spices instead of using salt or high-sodium seasonings or sauces.
- Choose low-sodium versions of soups, broths and sauces.
- Eliminate or cut the salt in half for most of your recipes. Many seasoning packets in easy-to-fix meals (e.g., macaroni and cheese) are high in sodium. Use ½ or less of the packet or substitute your own seasonings.
- Rinse canned vegetables with water to wash away extra sodium.

Add Fiber, Vitamins and Minerals

- Increase fiber by substituting whole wheat flour, oats or cornmeal for some of the flour in recipes. Substitute ½ of white flour in a recipe with whole wheat flour, or substitute ⅓ of white flour with oats.
- Add puréed fruits or vegetables in place of some of the water in recipes.
- Keep the peels on fruits and vegetables such as potatoes, carrots and apples.
- Add extra vegetables or grains such as rice, pasta or legumes to soups, sauces, salads and casseroles.
- Top a baked potato with steamed, fresh or stir-fried vegetables.

adding flavor the healthy way

Lowering Salt Intake

When it comes to health, sodium (salt) has drawn a considerable amount of attention because of its relationship to high blood pressure. High blood pressure is a leading risk factor for heart attack, stroke and kidney disease. Scientists have discovered that some people's blood pressure is very sensitive to excess sodium in the diet.

Because high blood pressure is such a serious health problem, the current U.S. Dietary Guidelines call for Americans to choose a diet moderate in salt and sodium. Most of the salt in the American diet comes from processed foods, however, not the saltshaker. Only about 15 percent of the sodium in the average diet is added in the kitchen or at the table. The top sources of salt in the diet include processed meats, prepackaged meals, fast foods, canned and dry soups, cheese, salted snack foods and certain condiments. The best way to learn how much sodium is in a food is to read the label. Foods that provide over 300 milligrams per serving are particularly high in sodium. For a single food item to carry the term "healthy" on the label, it must contain 360 or fewer milligrams of sodium per serving. Here are some foods particularly high in sodium.

- Canned and dry soups—1 cup contains 600-1,300 milligrams.
- Prepackaged meals (i.e., frozen dinners)—8 ounces contain 500-1,570 milligrams.
- Soy sauce—1 tablespoon contains 1,030 milligrams.
- Salted popcorn—2½ cups contain 330 milligrams.
- Processed cheese and cheese spreads—1 ounce contains 340-450 milligrams.
- Cured ham—3 ounces contain 1,025 milligrams.

While we're born with a preference for sweet tastes, salt is an acquired taste. Many people find that after cutting down on salt, many foods that they used to enjoy taste too salty. Cut down gradually to give your taste buds time to adapt. To be sure you consume no more than 2,400 milligrams of sodium per day, try these helpful tips.

- Choose foods that are naturally low in sodium, such as fresh fruits and vegetables.
- Break the habit of adding salt during cooking—there's no reason to salt cooking water—or at the table.
- Rinse canned meats, legumes and vegetables under cold water to remove excess salt.
- Eat a variety of foods during a single meal to stimulate the taste buds.
- Eat meals slowly and savor the flavor and aroma of each bite.
- Cut the salt called for in most recipes by half (or more).
- For meals with dried seasoning packets, use half or less of the packet to cut down on the sodium.
- Learn to season foods with herbs, spices, fruit juice and flavored vinegars.
- Limit processed meats such as ham, bacon, hot dogs and lunch meats.
- Limit high-salt condiments such as soy sauce, steak sauce, barbecue sauce, mustard and ketchup.
- Buy reduced-salt or low-salt snack foods.
- Limit consumption of olives, pickles, relishes and many salad dressings which are loaded with salt.

- When eating out, ask for meals to be prepared with less salt, ask for sauces to be served on the side and avoid using the saltshaker.

Herbs and Spices

Adding herbs, spices or other flavorings is a great way to make tasty dishes that are low in sodium. You'll have to experiment to find out what works best for you. Here are some tips on using and storing herbs and spices.

- Read the label; some premixed spices contain salt.
- Store herbs and spices in a cool, dark place and in tight containers. Avoid heat, moisture and light.
- Date dry herbs and spices when you buy them; shelf life is about one year.
- Test the freshness of herbs by rubbing them between your fingers and checking the aroma.
- Crumbling dry herbs between your fingers before using releases more flavor.
- Liquid brings out the flavor of dried herbs and spices.
- If you use fresh herbs, store them in a plastic bag in the refrigerator. Before using, wash and pat dry.
- For soups and stews—dishes that have to cook awhile—add herbs and spices toward the end of cooking.
- For chilled dishes or meats, the earlier you add the herbs and spices the better the flavor.
- When trying new herbs and spices, add them gradually to the dish— you can always add more.

Seasoning Ideas for Meat and Vegetables

Beef	Bay leaf, dry mustard, marjoram, nutmeg, onion, pepper, sage, thyme
Fish	Curry powder, dill, dry mustard, lemon juice, marjoram, paprika, pepper
Poultry	Ginger, marjoram, oregano, paprika, rosemary, sage, tarragon, sage, thyme
Carrots	Cinnamon, cloves, marjoram, nutmeg, rosemary, sage
Corn	Cumin, curry powder, green pepper, onion, paprika, parsley
Green beans	Dill, curry powder, lemon juice, marjoram, oregano, tarragon, thyme
Peas	Basil, dill, ginger, marjoram, onion, parsley, sage
Potatoes	Basil, dill, garlic, onion, paprika, parsley, rosemary, sage
Squash	Allspice, basil, cinnamon, curry powder, ginger, marjoram, nutmeg, onion, rosemary, sage
Tomatoes	Basil, bay leaf, dill, marjoram, onion, oregano, parsley, pepper, thyme

convenience foods—
making the most of your time

Does life have you on the go? *Of course it does!* Our fast-paced lives require us to cook and eat on the run. Fortunately, grocery store aisles are filled with convenience foods of all types—frozen dinners, canned soups, ready-to-eat cereals—and they come in all types of packages—jars, cans, bottles, boxes and bags. These foods save time in our busy lives, but they can also be high in calories, fat, cholesterol, added sugars and sodium.

Don't let busyness become a roadblock to achieving and maintaining a healthy weight and following a nutritious eating plan. The keys to healthy nutrition are balance, moderation and variety, even in convenience foods.

Reading Labels

The most popular trend in convenience foods over the last several years is the introduction of *low-fat* foods. Low-fat versions of our favorite foods are everywhere. Recently one shopper was quoted as saying, "There's low fat, no fat, fat free, nonfat and 95 percent fat free—I spent half the morning at the grocery store just looking at brownie labels!" You may feel the same way. You would think with all the low-fat foods available, Americans would be losing pounds by the truckload. However, surveys show that Americans are gaining more weight than ever. There's one important thing to keep in mind: *Low fat doesn't necessarily mean low calorie!*

Product	Calories	Product	Calories
Chocolate cream-filled cookie	53	Fat-free version	55
Fig bar	60	Fat-free version	70
Granola cereal	130	Reduced-fat version	110
Breakfast bar	120	Reduced-fat version	120
3-ounce bagel	150	Today's bigger version	400

Next time you shop, compare the calories on the low-fat foods you buy with the regular versions. Is there really a difference? Compare serving sizes too. Sometimes the difference in calories is actually due to the smaller size!

Choosing Healthy Convenience Foods

Dinners and single-item foods can fit into your daily balance of calories, fat, cholesterol, sodium, fiber and sugar. Use the following healthful guidelines to help you choose healthier convenience foods.

Look for Foods	Look for Clues on the Food Label	Know Your Daily Goal
Low in fat	3 or fewer grams of fat per serving	30 percent or less of total calories
Low in saturated fat	1 gram or less of saturated fat per serving	10 percent or less of total calories
Low in cholesterol	60 or fewer milligrams of cholesterol per serving	300 or fewer milligrams
Low in sodium	400 or fewer milligrams of sodium per serving	2,400 or fewer milligrams
High in fiber	2.5 or more grams of fiber per serving	25 to 30 grams of fiber
High in nutrients	10 percent or more of the RDI for one or more of the following: vitamin A, vitamin C, iron, calcium, protein and fiber	100 percent of the RDI

When choosing frozen dinners or entrees, use the following guidelines:

- Choose dinners that have fewer than 400 calories, 15 grams of fat, 5 grams of saturated fat and 800 milligrams of sodium.
- Choose entrees with fewer than 300 calories, 10 grams of fat and 4 grams of saturated fat.

Using Convenience Foods

- Compare food labels when shopping for convenience foods. Choose the food with the lowest saturated fat, cholesterol and sodium.
- When cooking packaged foods such as instant noodles or macaroni and cheese, lower the fat and calories by using less butter or margarine than the directions call for. Use half of the seasoning packet, or use your own seasonings, to lower the sodium content. Add your own fresh or frozen vegetables to add fiber, vitamins and minerals.
- When buying canned meat such as chicken, tuna or salmon, choose water-packed varieties instead of oil-packed.
- Choose breakfast cereals with terms such as "high fiber," "whole grain" or "bran" on the label. Cereals that are high in fiber (>2.5 grams per serving) and low in added sugar are good choices.
- Canned or frozen fruits and vegetables are good choices, but watch out for sodium and added fats. Rinse vegetables, beans and canned meats with water

to reduce the sodium content. Avoid canned and frozen vegetables with high-fat sauces.

- Limit use of frozen dinners and entrees with breaded or fried meats and vegetables.
- Buy prepackaged salads that contain an assortment of lettuce and other fresh vegetables. Be wary of salads that come with their own dressings and croutons, which are high in fat.
- Increase nutrients by balancing out your meal with a piece of fruit and a low-fat dairy product such as nonfat milk.
- Prepare your own healthy convenience foods by cooking your own recipes and freezing the leftovers in individual servings. Freezer bags and a variety of plastic containers make it convenient for you to store and reheat your meals.

meatless meals

For many people, meat is part of their daily meal plan. Unfortunately, meat is at the top of the list of foods that contribute the most calories, fat, saturated fat and cholesterol to the American diet. You don't have to eat meat every day to meet your body's nutritional needs. Research shows that an eating plan high in fruits, vegetables, whole grains and low-fat dairy products reduces the risk for many diseases, such as coronary heart disease, high blood pressure, diabetes and some forms of cancer. Eating a few meatless meals each week may be a healthy addition to your eating plan.

Reducing Meat Consumption

Most Americans eat much more protein than they need for good health. Keep in mind what counts as a serving (see page 160). Consider the typical portion sizes served in most restaurants and what you eat at home. As you'll probably realize, it's easy to eat more meat than you need.

One smart way to reduce your meat intake—and the fat and cholesterol that come with it—is to choose small portions of lean meats. Another way is to substitute other good sources of protein for meals that usually contain meat. Plant proteins can meet your body's daily needs, as long as you choose from a wide variety of protein-rich plant foods, such as whole grains, legumes, vegetables, low-fat dairy products, seeds and nuts. Remember, however, that some meatless sources of protein, such as cheese, nuts and seeds, can be high in calories and fat.

Caution: Besides meat, what other food provides the most calories, fat, saturated fat and cholesterol in the American diet? Cheese! It's common for people who are trying to eat less meat to substitute cheese instead. Watch out! Ounce for ounce, regular cheese has more fat and saturated fat than many cuts of meat and can be higher in cholesterol as well. Be sure to choose reduced-fat cheeses as often as possible. Choose cheeses with 3 to 5 grams of fat per ounce.

The legume family—beans, peas, lentils and soybeans—provides a good source of protein. Legumes are also good sources of carbohydrates, B vitamins and many other essential vitamins and minerals. They're a great source of soluble fiber, which helps lower blood cholesterol levels. Soy products, such as tofu, are especially good substitutes for animal proteins. Use legumes as the main part of any meal or add them to dishes such as soups, sauces and casseroles that typically call for meat. Choose any variety you like—kidney beans, navy beans, black beans, peas and lentils—and in any form—dried, canned, fresh or frozen.

Choosing Alternatives
To help get you started, here are some suggestions for meatless meals.

- Vegetarian pizza: Instead of meats, pile on the vegetables.
- Spaghetti with meatless sauce: Add beans or other vegetables to the sauce instead of meat.
- Casseroles: Use beans, whole grains or extra vegetables for some or all of the meat in the recipe.
- Bean burrito: Avoid beans refried in lard, and go easy on the cheese.
- Vegetarian soups: Replace the meat in soups with beans or whole grains, such as rice or pasta.
- Salads: Use beans, such as kidney or garbanzo, or low-fat cottage cheese instead of meat toppings.

Dining In or Out

Try some of these helpful ideas for meatless meals, or come up with your own.

Breakfast

- Select whole-grain, ready-to-eat cereal and nonfat milk.
- Choose whole-grain toast, English muffin, bagel or toaster waffle with jam or jelly. Add nonfat cream cheese or a little peanut butter as a source of protein.
- Low-fat yogurt is a great source of protein, calcium and other nutrients.

Lunch or Dinner

- Eat fresh vegetable salad, but go easy on the cheese. Add beans, peas, other legumes, nuts and seeds to boost protein, vitamins and minerals.
- Choose broth-based instead of cream-based meatless soups. Rice, pasta and other grains such as barley or tabouli are good substitutes for meat in many soups.
- Vegetable sandwiches are a good choice, but watch out for cheese and high-fat spreads such as cream cheese or mayonnaise. Try a vegetarian burger for a change of pace. These are usually made with whole grains, soy protein and other vegetables. They're lower in calories, fat and cholesterol than the traditional burger. Experiment until you find one you like.
- Prepare stir-fry with legumes, tofu or extra vegetables instead of meat.

Other Tips for Meatless Meals

- Choose restaurants with vegetarian choices; many ethnic cuisines offer meatless dishes.
- Order salads, soups, breads and fruits if a restaurant doesn't offer meatless dishes.
- When traveling, call the airline at least 48 hours in advance to request a meatless meal.

understanding portion control

Serving sizes may be one of the biggest factors causing the rising rate of obesity in this country. When it comes to food these days, bigger is better! There are "Super Meal Deals," "Super Size" and "50% More," and in many restaurants one meal is sometimes big enough to feed a family. Even too much of the right foods can make you gain weight. Learning appropriate portion sizes for different foods may be one of the most important skills you can learn when it comes to achieving and maintaining your healthy weight. It's a skill that takes time and practice to develop.

Mastering Portion Control

- **Use the right tools.** Make sure you use measuring cups and spoons and a food scale to help you learn about the portion sizes you eat. These tools allow you to compare what you *really* eat with what you *should* eat. Measure all the foods you eat to learn about common servings.
- **Try eating with smaller plates and bowls.** This will help you avoid serving portions that are too large. It also makes smaller portions look bigger.
- **Cut foods, such as meat, into smaller pieces.** This also gives the appearance of more food and can help the meal last longer.
- **Buy meats and cheese that are already cut in appropriate serving sizes.**
- **Get out of the habit of eating everything on your plate, especially at restaurants.** Learn to stop eating before you're full; it's okay to leave some food behind. It's also okay to split a meal with a companion.

Controlling Meat, Poultry and Fish Portions

One of the areas in which calories can easily add up unnoticed is the meat group. The recommended serving size for meat is three ounces. Unfortunately, we've gotten used to eating two to three times this amount. This is especially challenging when eating in restaurants. The average portion of meat served when dining out is 6 to 10 ounces. Remember, too, that restaurants don't always offer the leanest cuts of meat. With all of this in mind, it is a good idea to learn how to estimate a 3-ounce portion of meat.

3 OUNCES OF
MEAT, POULTRY
OR FISH =

¼ OF THE PLATE

COMPLEX
CARBOHYDRATES

COMPLEX
CARBOHYDRATES
STARCH=
¼ OF THE PLATE

VEGETABLES & FRUIT=
½ OF THE PLATE

• **Dinner-plate rule**—Imagine a standard dinner plate divided in quarters. Your meat serving should only fill one quarter of your plate. This means the other three-quarters should consist of complex carbohydrates—one-fourth starch and one-half vegetables/fruit.

• **Deck of cards rule**—An old favorite when trying to estimate 3-ounce portions of meat. A 3-ounce portion of meat should be no thicker and no wider than a standard deck of cards (or about the size of an audiocassette).

• **Lady's palm rule**—Three ounces of meat should fit nicely in the palm of an average-sized lady's hand.

• **Checkbook rule**—Three ounces of grilled fish is the size of a checkbook.

• **Eyeball rule**—This is a simple rule of thumb that is easy to apply—if it looks too big, it probably is!

When grocery shopping, keep in mind that chicken breasts are typically closer to 5 or 6 ounces each. Individual filet mignons, although they look small, are at least 6- to 8-ounce portions. It's a good idea to plan on cutting these portions in half before preparing. Eating a couple of ounces more than you should can add at least 100 calories!

Shortcuts for Estimating Portion Sizes

The key to moderation is controlling portion size. To achieve and maintain a healthy weight, learn to put into practice the concepts of "serving size." Use measuring cups, spoons and scales until you know appropriate portion sizes by heart. Following are some practical examples from the American Dietetics Association to help you estimate portion sizes when these tools aren't available:

• A medium potato should be the size of a computer mouse.
• An average bagel should be the size of a hockey puck.
• A cup of fruit is the size of a baseball.
• A cup of lettuce is four leaves.
• One ounce of cheese is the size of four dice.
• One ounce of snack foods, such as pretzels, is one handful.

DINING ON THE GO

the anytime, anywhere restaurant guide

Eating out is a great way to spend time with family and friends and enjoy good food. Believe it or not, you can dine out without blowing your healthy eating plan! The key is having a plan and sticking with it.

Check Out What's on the Menu

Menus are full of food clues if you know what to look for. Here is a list of terms often used in menus.

Less Fat	More fat
Baked or broiled	Fried
Poached	Breaded
Grilled	Sautéed (in butter or oil)
Tomato sauce	Alfredo or cream sauce
Roasted	Casserole
Steamed	Prime

Big portions are a problem when eating out. Almost any restaurant meal can be a good choice if you don't eat all of it. The key to controlling portions is to have a plan before you order. Try the following helpful tips:

- Choose single items and side dishes rather than complete meals.
- Ask for a to-go box before you eat your meal. Choose what you need and immediately box the rest.

- Share a dish with a companion or plan to eat smaller portions of dishes that are higher in calories, fat and sugar.

Healthy Choices for Any Meal

A Healthy Start

- Choose toast, small (or half) bagel or English muffin with a small amount of margarine or low-fat cream cheese and jam or jelly. Add nonfat milk and fruit or fruit juice to balance out your meal.
- Cold or hot cereals with nonfat milk are a great start to any day. Top with fresh or dried fruit for added nutrition. Choose wholesome cereals with little or no added sugar and three or more grams of fiber.
- Limit eggs (two or three each week), bacon, sausage, fried potatoes, biscuits, croissants and sweet rolls. Muffins can be high in calories, fat and sugar.

Midday Munching

- Broth-based soups and fresh salads with dressing on the side make a great noontime choice. Watch out for cream-based soups and potato, macaroni, tuna or chicken salads which are made with mayonnaise.
- Choose sandwiches with grilled chicken, lean roast beef, turkey or ham. Some deli-style sandwiches pack on the meat; ask for more vegetables instead. Order mustard or low-fat spreads instead of mayonnaise.
- Limit French fries, onion rings and chips. Ask that they be left off your plate or substitute a baked potato, fruit or vegetables. Burgers and hot dogs are okay occasionally, but avoid the deluxe versions.

A Night Out

- Choose baked, broiled or grilled chicken (without the skin), fish or small portions of other lean meats. Limit fried and prime cuts of meat and heavy sauces.
- Pastas with tomato-based sauces and fresh vegetables are good choices. Limit cream- or cheese-based sauces. When you order, ask that the sauce be served on the side.
- Start your meal with a fresh salad and broth-based soup to help control your appetite. Better yet, when you know you are dining out, eat a piece of fruit or drink a glass of nonfat milk before you go.

Satisfy Your Sweet Tooth

- First, ask yourself if you're really hungry. If you're not, save the dessert for another time. If you are hungry, the best choices include fresh fruit, sorbet, frozen yogurt, sherbet or angel food cake with a fruit topping.
- Desserts aren't always off-limits, just keep your overall goals in mind. If you know ahead of time that you want dessert, plan to split your favorite treat with a companion. Another option is to eat slowly and to eat only a few bites.

More Survival Tips

- When eating out with family and friends, tell them in advance that you plan to eat healthy. Order what you know is best for you, and don't allow yourself to be tempted by others.
- If you know a meal will be high in calories and fat, choose more healthy foods during the rest of the day. Don't skip any meals!
- When eating at a buffet, plan in advance to choose healthier foods. Fill up on low-fat items such as fruits, vegetables, low-fat breads and crackers and lean meats.
- When eating out, you can burn off a few extra calories by parking your car a few blocks away and walking. Make a plan to go for a walk before or after eating.

dining asian style

Asian restaurants have become an American favorite. With a variety of foods, cooking styles and atmospheres, they offer both enjoyable and healthful dining. Asian restaurants often use low-fat cooking methods and lean meats, fresh vegetables, rice and noodles. However, these same nutritious foods are often deep-fried or stir-fried and served with high-sodium sauces. Add in the typically large portions and an egg roll, and a single meal can easily top 1,500 calories.

What to Order

With the diversity of Asian cuisine—Chinese, Japanese, Thai, Korean and Vietnamese—and cooking styles, it's important to know how to read menus. The following chart of the most common menu items and terms will aid you in choosing wisely. Choose low-fat items more often and high-fat and high-sodium items less often.

Low in Fat	High in Fat	High in Sodium
Barbecued	Coconut milk	Black bean sauce
Bean curd	Duck	Hoisin sauce
Braised	Egg rolls	Miso sauce
Roasted or grilled	Fried or crispy	Most soups
Simmered	Fried rice or noodles	Oyster sauce
Steamed	Peanuts or cashews	Pickled
Stir-fried	Tempura	Soy sauce
Water chestnuts	Wonton	Teriyaki sauce

Did You Know?

- **Some Asian sauces, such as sweet-and-sour and plum sauce, are actually low in fat, calories and sodium.** The problem is that dishes served with these sauces often consist of deep-fried meats.
- **A tablespoon of soy sauce has nearly 1,000 milligrams of sodium**—almost half of the recommended daily intake of 2,400 milligrams.
- **While Asian cuisine uses lots of vegetables, salads are somewhat unusual.** The exceptions are Thai and Vietnamese cuisine, which offer a variety of salads, including garden salads.
- **The trendy Japanese sushi—a combination of raw fish, vinegared rice and often seaweed—is actually low in fat, calories and sodium, depending on the dipping sauce.**

Healthy Choices for Any Occasion

Appetizers and Soups

Traditional appetizers such as egg rolls, wonton and fried shrimp are high in calories and fat. Ask if the restaurant offers steamed spring rolls or steamed dumplings instead. If you choose the egg roll, eat only the inside.

Many Asian soups, such as hot-and-sour and egg-drop, offer a great way to start a meal. These broth-based soups are low in calories and fat.

The Main Meal

Asian dishes are usually served in large portions—enough for at least two people. Remember a serving of rice is one-half of a cup! Ask for a to-go box before your meal, and store away the extra portions for another meal. It's usually a good idea to order fewer dishes than people and then share them family style.

Choose the following dishes more often:

✓ Dishes with steamed rice or noodles.

✓ Steamed fish, stir-fried chicken or other lean meats.

✓ Stir-fried dishes with fresh vegetables such as broccoli, cabbage, carrots, water chestnuts, mushrooms and sprouts. Try tofu!

✓ For dessert, have the fortune cookie if you want. Coconut desserts can be high in fat and calories.

Choose the following dishes less often:

✓ Fried rice, noodles, egg rolls and wonton.

✓ Breaded and fried meats found in tempura or sweet-and-sour sauce. Ask how the meat is prepared before ordering.

✓ Dishes with cashews or peanuts—ask that the amount of nuts be cut in half.

More Helpful Tips

- **Let family or friends who are dining with you know that you plan to eat healthy.** Don't let what others order change your plans for choosing nutritious low-fat and low-calorie foods.

- **Become familiar with a few restaurants you enjoy where you know you can order healthy foods.** Learn to make special requests, such as substituting steamed rice for fried rice. Ask that your meal be prepared with less oil or fewer added fats. Avoid restaurants or foods that can tempt you from your plan.

- **If you order an item that is higher in fat, balance it with a low-fat choice,** such as steamed rice or steamed vegetables.

- **Ask that stir-fry and other dishes be cooked with very little oil.**

- **Be careful when eating Asian food buffet style.** Plan to make healthy choices and select reasonable portions.

- **When eating take-out food at home, serve what you need on a plate and store the rest.**

dining *delizioso!*

Italian food is an American favorite! Almost everyone has a favorite little Italian restaurant. Typically serving good food and having quaint atmospheres, they are a great place to fellowship with family and friends. Italian food offers many healthy choices. Fresh breads, pastas and tomato-based sauces are great choices on any eating plan. But depending on how they're prepared, these same foods can be less-healthy choices: garlic bread with butter and cheese, pastas cooked in oil or covered with cheese, cream-based sauces and large portions. Add the cheesecake, and you can easily exceed a day's worth of calories.

A Taste of Italy

You may not speak Italian, but you can learn how to read the menu. Learn the following common terms to help you make more-healthful choices:

Low in Fat	High in Fat
Baked, broiled or roasted	*Alfredo*—butter or cheese sauces
Marinara—tomato-based sauces	Cheese- or meat-filled pastas
Marsala or *cacciatore*	*Crema*—cream-based sauces
Minestrone	*Fritto*—fried
Primavera	Garlic bread
Red or white clam sauce	*Parmigiana*

Note: Just because it's green doesn't mean it's low fat! *Pesto*, made with basil, olive oil, pine nuts and grated cheese, is generally high in fat and calories. Use it carefully!

Healthy Choices for Any Occasion

Appetizers
How does hot garlic bread sound? Be careful—a couple of slices can add up to 500 calories! Ask that your waiter not bring the garlic bread to the table, or plan to split a piece with a companion. Dipping your bread in olive oil also adds calories. Ask for bread without the butter, or have breadsticks instead.

Start your meal with minestrone soup or gazpacho and a salad with dressing on the side. You can even make these your main meal. A Caesar salad with eggs, creamy dressing, grated cheese and croutons is generally high in fat and calories. Do you enjoy antipasto? Antipasto with seafood and marinated vegetables is usually your best choice. Watch out for antipasto with lots of cheese, fried vegetables, meats and olives, all of which can be high in calories, sodium and fat.

The Main Meal

Italian portions are often two to three times more than you need. Remember a serving of pasta is a half cup! Ask for a to-go box before your meal and keep the extra portions for another day, or consider splitting a dish with a companion.

Choose the following dishes more often:
- ✓ Grilled chicken breast or veal with marsala or cacciatore.
- ✓ Pasta with marinara or pasta primavera (pasta with vegetables).
- ✓ Clam sauce.

Choose the following dishes less often:
- ✓ Lasagna or cheese-filled pasta (ravioli, cannelloni and manicotti)
- ✓ Italian sausage, pancetta (bacon) or prosciutto (ham).
- ✓ Eggplant or veal parmigiana—breaded or fried.

Pizza

Pizza can be a healthy choice. Here are some tips for ordering.

- **Choose a thin crust instead of thick-crust or deep-dish pizza.**
- **Ask that your pizza be prepared with less cheese (or even no cheese).**
- **Select vegetables as toppings instead of high-fat and high-sodium meats.**
- **Limit yourself to one or two pieces.** For added variety, eat a salad instead of an extra piece.

More Helpful Tips

- **Make a plan and stick with it.** Remember your goal of reaching or maintaining a healthy weight.

- **Let family or friends who are dining with you know that you plan to eat healthy.** Don't let what others order change your plans for choosing nutritious low-fat and low-calorie foods.
- **Become familiar with a few restaurants you enjoy where you know you can order healthy foods.** Learn to make special requests, such as substituting tomato-based sauces for cream- or cheese-based sauces. Ask that your meal be prepared with less oil or butter. Avoid restaurants and foods that can tempt you to stray from your plan.
- **When eating take-out food at home, serve what you need on a plate and store the rest.**

dining south-of-the-border style

Mexican food is known for its hot and spicy flavors. Dining south of the border is also popular for its festive atmosphere. Mexican restaurants offer good times and good food. You might think that Mexican food is off-limits. Actually, the staples of Mexican cuisine offer nutritious choices: chicken and other lean meats, tortillas, beans, rice and salsa. Of course, many also offer less-healthy choices such as fried tortillas, refried beans, too much cheese, high-fat dips and sauces and portions that are too large. Be careful or your food fiesta can easily exceed a whole day's worth of calories and fat!

Menu Lingo
To make healthy choices, you must first learn to read the menu.

Low in Fat	High in Fat
Baked, broiled, simmered or *asada* (grilled)	*Chili con queso* (cheese sauce)
Fajitas (grilled meat and soft tortillas)	*Chorizo* (sausage)
Picante sauce or salsa	Fried or crispy
Salsa verde (green sauce)	Guacamole and sour cream
Veracruz or *ranchero* (tomato-based) sauces	Refried, often with lard

Healthy Choices

Appetizers

How do hot chips with fresh salsa or chili con queso sound? It's easy to consume 500 calories or more before your meal arrives. Plan ahead to limit the number of chips you will eat (5 to 8 chips are around 100 calories). Better yet, ask that chips not be brought to your table. Ask for steamed corn tortillas instead.

Tortilla or bean soup and a salad are a healthy start to your meal—they can even be the whole meal! Ask for the salad dressing, guacamole and sour cream to be served on the side. Salsa makes a nutritious no-fat dressing. Watch out for taco salad though—particularly if it's served in a tortilla shell.

The Main Meal

Mexican dinners tend to be large. Avoid combination or deluxe plates, and order a la carte or side orders instead. Another option is to split a combination plate with a companion.

Choose the following dishes more often:
- ✓ Grilled chicken breast with rice and vegetables.
- ✓ Fajitas with grilled chicken or lean meat, but watch out for cheese, guacamole and sour cream; ask for extra lettuce, tomatoes and salsa instead.
- ✓ Chicken enchiladas with red or green (*verde*) sauce; hold the sour cream.
- ✓ Bean or chicken burritos made with a soft (not fried) tortilla. Request the amount of cheese to be cut in half.

Choose the following dishes less often:
- ✓ Tacos, chalupas and flautas.
- ✓ Cheese enchiladas or enchiladas with cheese or cream sauce.
- ✓ *Carnitas* (fried beef or pork) or chorizo.
- ✓ Fried burrito or *chimichanga*.

More Helpful Tips

- **Make a plan and stick with it.** Remember your goal of reaching or maintaining a healthy weight.

- Let family or friends who are dining with you know that you plan to eat healthy. Don't let what others order change your plans for choosing nutritious low-fat and low-calorie foods.
- Become familiar with a few restaurants you enjoy where you know you can order healthy foods.
- Order a side of Mexican rice and pinto or black beans—instead of refried beans—with your main item.
- Avoid restaurants or foods that can tempt you from your plan.
- Order a la carte items. This allows you to pick and choose the foods that are healthiest and that you enjoy.
- Watch portion sizes. Ask for a to-go box before your meal or split your meal with a companion.
- When eating take-out food at home, serve what you need on a plate and store the rest.

No matter whether it's traditional Mexican cuisine, Tex-Mex or Mexican-American, you can enjoy a healthful meal when eating south of the border. Simply follow four simple guidelines: Have a plan; know how to find healthful choices; order wisely; and eat what you know is best for you.

life in the fast-food lane

Eating in the fast-food lane has become a way of life for many of us. Life has us on the go, so we have to eat on the go. Why do people choose to eat fast foods? *Taste, convenience* and *price* top the list. These reasons are important, but good nutrition and health should be at the top of your list.

Fast-Food Fare

What foods do you think of when you think fast food: burgers and fries, fried chicken, tacos and burritos, soft drinks? A fast-food meal can easily top 1,000 calories and give you a day's worth of fat, cholesterol and sodium. Believe it or not, you can also make healthy fast-food choices. Today, most fast-food restaurants offer a variety of foods such as grilled chicken, salads, baked potatoes and deli-style sandwiches. Of course, fresh fruits and vegetables are hard to find. The key is to plan ahead and be prepared to make healthy choices. Look for ways to trim fat, cut calories and add variety whenever you can. Always keep your goals of a healthy weight and good nutrition in mind. Here are some helpful tips—pick the ones that will work best for you.

Eating on the Go

- **Order individual items rather than the special meal deal.** One item that is higher in calories and fat may be okay, but add fries and a soft drink and you may double the calories and fat.
- **Watch out for words such as "deluxe," "supersize" or "jumbo."** Order the regular or small size instead. A single slice of cheese on a small burger adds calcium. Think nutrition—add the cheese and cut the fries.
- **Choose sandwiches with grilled chicken or fish, or lean roast beef, turkey or ham.** Ask for low-fat toppings such as mustard or low-fat salad dressing instead of mayonnaise or special sauce.
- **If you're having fast food for one meal, choose healthier foods the rest of the day.** Don't forget your fruits and vegetables. You can even carry a piece of fruit with you to eat with your meal.

Lettuce Works

- **Beware—salads can have more calories, fat and sodium than a burger and fries!** Limit items such as cheese, croutons, bacon, eggs, nuts and creamy salad dressings. Add more vegetables instead.
- **Always order salad dressing on the side.** Use the low-fat dressing whenever possible. Salsa and low-fat cottage cheese are also good choices. Add flavor with fresh fruits, peppers and other vegetables.
- **Limit special salads such as potato, macaroni, tuna and chicken.** These salads are often made with mayonnaise or high-fat salad dressing. Choose coleslaw or bean salad made with vinaigrette instead.

Potato Toppings

- **Plain baked potatoes are low in calories and fat and are a good source of fiber and vitamin C.** Limit toppings such as butter, cheese, bacon and sour cream.
- **Healthier choices include small amounts of margarine and low-fat sour cream.** Other good toppings include low-fat cottage cheese, plain yogurt and salsa. Pack on the nutrition by adding lots of fresh vegetables.

Fast-Food Olé

- Choose grilled chicken (without the skin), beans or vegetables instead of beef or cheese on tostados, tacos or burritos. Ask for your bean burrito to be prepared with less cheese. Order soft tortillas rather than fried.
- Go easy on—or abstain from—cheese, sour cream and guacamole. Add more lettuce, tomatoes and salsa.

The Orient Express

- Asian takeout is one fast-food option that offers a variety of vegetables. Watch out, however, portion sizes can be large! Make a plan to split a dish with a companion or save some for another meal.
- Ask before you order. Many Asian dishes include fried meats. Order steamed rice instead of fried rice, forego the fried egg roll and ask for extra vegetables.

The Pizza Plan

- Choose thin crust over thick crust or deep dish.
- Avoid meats such as ground beef and pepperoni. These meats are higher in fat and sodium. Instead, ask for extra tomato sauce, fresh vegetables and less cheese.
- Limit yourself to one or two slices.
- Order a salad. A healthy salad will add variety and nutrition to your meal.

Drink Up

- Choose low-fat milk or natural fruit juice to drink. This will boost the nutrition of any fast-food meal. Water is always a good choice!
- Remember that some milk shakes can equal the calories and fat of an entire meal. Keep this in mind, and cut back in other areas if you order the shake.

A Healthy Beginning

- If breakfast is most often your fast-food meal, choose a plain bagel, toast or English muffin with jelly, jam or low-fat cream cheese. Skip the croissant and biscuits, which are high in fat and calories.
- Cold or hot cereals with nonfat milk, pancakes without butter or plain scrambled eggs are also good choices. Limit high-fat meats such as bacon and sausage and watch out for fried potatoes.

nutrition while traveling

Whether traveling for business or pleasure, eating healthy on the road can be difficult. The secret is *getting away* without *getting back* all the weight you've worked so hard *getting off*. With a little planning, you can keep on track when you travel.

How to Eat Healthy

Part of the enjoyment of traveling is the chance to try out new cuisine. When you travel, allow yourself to enjoy new foods. A *few* choices that are higher in fat, sugar and calories are okay.

The key is to plan ahead how you want to eat while traveling and stick to it. Get support from your traveling companions. Let them know that you plan to eat healthy. It's much easier to make healthy choices when you have the support of others. Plus, you might be a positive influence on them!

On the Road

- **Pack your own snacks.** Good choices include bagels, fresh or dried fruits, raw vegetables, low-fat crackers, rice cakes, pretzels and cereal bars. By having your own snacks with you, you can avoid becoming too hungry and then overeating the first chance you get.
- **Eat a healthy meal before you hit the road.** Filling up before you leave will help you avoid making less healthful choices while on the road.
- **Pack a cooler.** Take along sandwiches, fruits, vegetables, low-fat yogurt and healthy beverages such as water, juice and low-fat milk.
- **When eating at fast-food restaurants, avoid fried foods and supersized or deluxe meals.** Choose regular-sized portions and choose grilled chicken or other lean-meat sandwiches, baked potatoes (but easy on the cheese!) and fresh salads.
- **Stop regularly for a little physical activity,** such as stretching and a short walk—every little bit helps!

In the Air

- **Don't eat the airline meal just because it's offered.** Ask yourself if you're hungry. What are your meal plans when you arrive? If you're not hungry or you're planning to eat when you arrive, save the calories. Instead, ask for milk or juice and a snack to curb your appetite.

- Call at least 48 hours in advance to request a special meal: low-fat, low-cholesterol or vegetarian.
- Drinking water is the best choice for staying hydrated in the pressurized environment. You should also choose fruit or vegetable juice, low-fat milk or water instead of soft drinks or other beverages.
- Bring your own food in a carry-on bag. Good choices include fresh and dried fruit, ready-to-eat cereals, bagels, crackers and low-fat cheese.
- Eat a healthy meal or snack before you arrive at the airport or board the airplane.
- Walk around the airport. This is a good idea not only for the exercise, but it also gives you the opportunity to stake out healthy food options.
- When the "fasten seat belt" sign goes off, get up and walk up and down the aisle every 20 minutes or so.

Out on the Town

- Choose restaurants wisely. You can call the restaurant ahead of time to check out the menu. Ask if they prepare food to order or accept special requests.
- Watch out for those large portions. Try to choose smaller portions or share larger portions with a companion. Three ounces of meat is about the size of a deck of playing cards.
- Don't skip meals to save up for that special meal. Balance out a meal higher in fat and calories by making healthier choices during the day.
- If you eat dessert, share it with a companion or take only a few bites.
- Beware of buffets. Load up on fresh fruits, vegetables and other low-fat choices. Don't load up your plate just because it's "all you can eat." Rather than trying all the foods, pick one or two of your favorites and keep your portions small.
- Eating smaller portions is a good way to enjoy a variety of foods. Balance less healthy choices with better choices such as fresh fruits, vegetables and whole-grain foods.
- When dining in foreign countries, you may need to avoid raw fruits and vegetables, raw or partly cooked meats and tap water. A good rule to remember: If it's been boiled, cooked, bottled or peeled, it's probably okay.

More Helpful Tips

- **Stay at hotels and resorts that offer healthy dining options.**
- **Start each day with a healthy breakfast.** Fresh fruit, toast, a bagel or English muffin with jam; hot or cold cereal; and low-fat yogurt are good choices. Fresh-squeezed juice and low-fat or nonfat milk are good beverage choices. Limit your intake of eggs, sausage, bacon, sweet rolls, donuts, croissants and fried potatoes.
- **Carry snacks with you to business meetings or while sightseeing.** Try to avoid becoming overly hungry. If you wait too long between meals, you're more likely to overeat or make less healthy choices.
- **Make time for physical activity.**

Watch for Hidden Fats

When eating away from home, it can be difficult to estimate how much fat is in a meal. It's important to estimate hidden fats in food because extra calories can add up quickly. Just one teaspoon of oil or one tablespoon of salad dressing has 5 grams of fat and 45 calories. Considering that a ladle of dressing at most salad bars is three or four tablespoons, it's easy to see how fat calories can add up!

The best way to control hidden fats when eating out is to ask that foods be prepared without added fats and that salad dressing, gravies and sauces be served on the side.

take time for a healthy lunch

Do you take time for lunch? Our busy lifestyles often lead to lunch on the run. For many, lunch is a popular social time rather than a time to nourish the body. Some of us are so busy we don't even take time for lunch.

The most popular lunchtime fares are sandwiches, hamburgers and salads. The truth of the matter is that traditional sandwiches and salads may not be any lower in fat and calories than the fast-food burger!

Avoiding lunch leads to fatigue, hunger and overeating later in the day or night. Extreme hunger can also lead to cravings for junk food and binge eating. On the positive side, a nutritious lunch can give your body the fuel it needs to meet the physical and mental demands of the rest of the day. Lunchtime can also offer a much-needed break after a hard morning of work. A light nutritious meal plus 10 to 20 minutes of moderate activity during the lunch hour is a great way to achieve good health and a healthy weight. Eating too much fat, calories and sugar may do you in for the rest of the day.

Excuses for Not Eating a Healthy Lunch

- **I don't have time!** Even if you can't stop for a relaxing lunch break, you can take a few minutes to eat some nutritious foods. It's easy to eat a sandwich, cheese and crackers, yogurt or fresh fruit—if you have prepared ahead of time.
- **I don't need the calories!** This is *not* a good reason to skip lunch. Your body needs energy and nutrients throughout the day. Skipping meals only leads to overeating later in the day. With every meal you skip, you rob your body of important nutrients and sources for the energy needed to make it through the afternoon hours.

Examine your reasons for not eating a healthy lunch. What are some possible solutions? What are the benefits of eating a nutritious lunch? Begin making plans to make a nutritious lunch a regular part of your day.

Eating Out

Eating a healthy lunch is now easier than ever. Fast-food and other restaurants now offer several nutritious and low-fat options. Of course, most menus offer selections that are high in calories, fat and cholesterol, and low in fresh fruits, vegetables and whole grains. The key is to plan ahead and order what you know is best.

Best Bets for a Healthy Lunch

- A fresh salad with an assortment of colorful vegetables, low-fat dressing (*On the side, please!*), grilled chicken, grilled chicken sandwich (*Hold the mayo!*), bean and cheese burrito (*Go easy on the cheese and add extra lettuce and tomato!*), small hamburger or baked potato (*Toppings on the side!*) are all good choices. All these meals have fewer than 400 calories and 30 percent or less fat.
- Deli sandwiches can be a healthy choice. Choose lean meats such as turkey, ham or roast beef. Ask for mustard or light mayonnaise. Ask for less meat (usually half the typical serving), more lettuce, tomato and other vegetables, and whole-grain bread. Hold the chips or fries.

- Pizza can be a good choice if you choose carefully. Stick to vegetable pizza and ask for less cheese and more sauce and vegetables. Limit yourself to one or two slices of thin-crust pizza. Eat a salad too—with low-fat dressing on the side!
- Pick out three or four restaurants where you know you can get healthy foods. Suggest to friends and colleagues that you eat at these places when you eat out for lunch.

Worst Bets for a Healthy Lunch

- A hamburger and fries, a tuna-salad sandwich or a chicken Caesar salad can supply half of the fat and calories recommended for an entire day. The typical deli-style sandwich piled with meat, mayonnaise and cheese—and bacon if it's a club sandwich—is not any better.
- Is salad a healthy choice? It depends on what you put in/on it. A ladle of regular salad dressing contains four tablespoons—nearly 300 calories of fat or half of your recommended daily intake.
- Fried foods—french fries, fried chicken and fish, burgers, tacos, etc.—should not be a regular part of the lunchtime meal. Frying can double the fat and calories.
- Portion sizes can be two to three times what you need—split a meal with a companion or take some home to eat for another meal.

Packing Your Lunch

Packing a healthy lunch starts with planning. A healthy brown-bag lunch starts in the grocery store. Plan ahead to buy a variety of nutritious foods that you enjoy and are convenient for you to prepare and pack along. When preparing your lunch, remember the key principles of variety, balance and moderation.

- You'll need an assortment of plastic containers, plastic bags and maybe even a thermos. An insulated lunch bag or cooler can keep foods cool if you don't have access to a refrigerator.
- Canned and frozen fruits, vegetables and beans can be placed in individual-sized plastic containers. You can do the same with soups. Add your own seasonings when packing. Your meal is now ready to heat in a microwave when you're ready.
- Take along low-fat dairy foods. Milk can be kept cool in a thermos and yogurt can stay at room temperature for several hours. Mix canned fruit or fresh vegetables with cottage cheese in a plastic container.

- Keep plenty of your favorite fruits and vegetables on hand wherever you are. If they need cutting or peeling, do it the night before. Better yet, prepare them as soon as you come home from the grocery store. Store them away in plastic bags or containers so they're ready to go when you are.
- Make a sandwich with lean meat and fresh vegetables the night before. Place it in a sandwich container or plastic bag and it will be ready to go when you leave in the morning.
- Make lunch quick and easy by bringing leftovers. Most leftovers can be easily reheated in a microwave. When cooking at home, make extra portions and store the extras individually for a ready-to-serve lunch.
- Packing your own lunch also saves money; it's much cheaper to pack your own than to eat out. The savings over an entire year could pay for a health club membership or home exercise equipment!
- Always have enjoyable standbys when you find yourself short on time or choices. Dried and canned soups and fruits, crackers, peanut butter, oatmeal, cereal, bagels and energy bars can be kept on hand in a pantry or desk drawer for a quick and easy lunch anytime.

PHYSICAL FITNESS

the amazing 10-minute workout

No time, no fun and bo-or-or-ring! These are common reasons people give for not making physical activity a lifetime habit. Yet experts are making it harder and harder to come up with good excuses. The latest recommendations tell us that exercise doesn't have to be hard to be beneficial. Gone are the days when you had to exercise for at least 30 minutes at a certain heart rate to get the health and fitness benefits of aerobic exercise. What's the exercise prescription for today? "Something is better than nothing, and more is better than something."

The latest recommendations from groups such as the American Heart Association and the American College of Sports Medicine call for at least 30 minutes of moderate physical activity on as many days of the week as possible—preferably every day. The latest twist on this new recommendation is that the activity doesn't have to be done all at one time. Shorter amounts accumulated over the course of a day appear to offer the same health benefits as the more traditional 30 continuous minutes of exercise.

The Benefits of Shorter Workouts

Shorter workouts are easier to start and to stick with. It's easy to get burned out on exercise by doing too much too soon. Start slow and work your way up to longer sessions as your physical activity becomes a habit.

You may also be a person who just doesn't have 30 to 60 minutes to give at one time. Shorter workouts are easier to fit into your schedule and will help fight boredom by allowing more variety in your routine. They're also great for regular exercisers who occasionally miss or are unable to do their usual routine. When you miss or know you are going to miss a session, just slip in one or two of these shorter workouts wherever and whenever you can.

How to Do It

Are lack of time, lack of enjoyment and boredom among the reasons you have a hard time making exercise a part of your life? Whether you're a regular exerciser or just getting started, consider some of the following ideas for fitting 10-minute workouts into your day:

- Walking can be done anywhere, anytime. Think about times in your typical day when you can fit in a short, brisk walk.
- Get up 10 minutes earlier and fit in a quick walk before starting your day.
- Walk as part of your daily quiet time.
- Take 10-minute walking breaks at work.
- Arrive to work 10 minutes early and walk or climb the stairs.
- Take a 10-minute walk around the mall before stopping to shop.
- Walk your dog for 10 minutes.
- Take the entire family out for a 10-minute walk before or after meals.
- Walk around the house during commercials or between shows—you'll easily get in 10 minutes.

Walking is not your only choice. Here are some other creative ideas.

- Pick up the pace when you're doing household chores: 10 minutes of vacuuming, washing the car or working in the yard add up over the course of a day. To get the benefit, however, you have to push the pace a bit. Turn on your favorite music to help keep you moving.
- Buy an exercise video and pop it in for 10 minutes.
- Do you have exercise equipment that's collecting dust? Pull it out and try a 10-minute routine instead of feeling like you have to stay on for 30 minutes or longer.
- Rather than just watching your kids play, spend 10 minutes playing with them: shoot baskets, throw a ball or Frisbee, kick a soccer ball, etc.
- Take 10-minute breaks at work and do calisthenics, strength training or stretching exercises.

Choose a few activities that you enjoy and can do for approximately 10 minutes at a time. Be creative—don't limit yourself to the traditional exercises. Whatever you choose to do, try to make it fun. Remember, the *E* in *exercise* is for *enjoyment!*

Once you've chosen a few activities, think of some times you can fit them into your day. Think about times in your day when you can be more active, such as when you watch television, shop, work around the house or take a break.

choosing a personal trainer

Working with a personal trainer is a great way to get your fitness program headed in the right direction. A personal trainer can give support, guidance and instruction in the pursuit of your aerobic, strength and flexibility goals. Making an appointment with a trainer is similar to joining an accountability group. The trainer holds clients accountable for a time slot, and the client carves out a specific time every day during which exercise is the priority.

Do I Need a Personal Trainer?
- Are you familiar with weight equipment and cardiovascular machines?
- Will it help you to have a professional design and supervise an individualized program?
- Will having a trainer help you achieve the goals you have set for yourself?
- Do you have special needs that require individual supervision?
- Are you more motivated to exercise if you have scheduled time to do so?

If you answered yes to any of these questions, a personal trainer may be right for you. You may want a trainer on a regular basis or only occasionally to update your exercise program and receive feedback on progress. Working with a personal trainer for a few sessions is often all it takes for some people to feel comfortable with an exercise program. For others a personal trainer is a great way to increase adherence to an exercise regimen.

Guidelines for Choosing a Personal Trainer

Following is a list of questions to ask the candidate you are considering as a personal trainer. In addition, note whether the trainer works in a fitness center, does in-home training or both.

- Does the trainer have a degree in a health-related field and a nationally accredited certification?
- Does he or she have liability insurance? Ask for proof of coverage.
- Does the trainer have at least two to three years of experience in the health and fitness field?
- Is he or she professional, punctual and personable?
- Does he or she have a strong background in the biomechanics and physiology of exercise?
- Is the trainer well read in current issues and trends in health and fitness (e.g., does he or she subscribe to professional journals or other publications)?
- Does the trainer know how to vary workout intensity in accordance with your personal needs?
- Does he or she keep records of your progress and review your results regularly?

If the candidate you are interviewing can answer yes to all of these questions, then you are well on your way to a positive personal training experience. Don't hesitate to ask for the names and phone numbers of other clients with goals similar to yours. Call to see if they were pleased with their workouts, if the trainer was punctual and prepared, and if they felt their individual needs were addressed. Finally, ask yourself if you could get along well with the trainer and whether or not he or she seems genuinely interested in helping you. If the trainer meets all your other prerequisites, this is the trainer to hire. Together, you and your trainer can determine your best route to better health and fitness.

Cautions

Red Flags	Did You Know?
Beware of a trainer whose degree or certification cannot be documented.	One does not have to have a degree or certification to become a personal trainer
Bodybuilders and other athletes don't automatically qualify as good personal trainers.	Some fitness centers and clubs require a degree and a nationally accredited certification for their trainers, but many don't.
Beware of someone who *only* knows how to prescribe a bodybuilding type of workout.	Some trainers are independent contractors, and some are employees of the fitness center.
Be wary of a trainer who can't verify proof of liability insurance.	A personal trainer can be very helpful when it's time to start or update an exercise program.
Watch out if a trainer doesn't use gradual methods to increase strength, aerobic conditioning and flexibility.	A good personal trainer will pay attention to your total fitness.
Beware of a trainer who does not have a 24-hour cancellation policy.	The American College of Sports Medicine, the American Council on Exercise, the National Strength and Conditioning Association and the National Academy of Sports Medicine are all accredited certifying bodies.

Signs of a Quality Trainer

A quality trainer will listen carefully to all of your concerns and questions. The trainer's goal should be to help you develop a program that is right for you— not one that's right for him or her! He or she should rely on scientifically and medically supported information on health and fitness and should refer you to a physician or a registered dietitian in the event that specific health questions arise or specific dietary guidelines are requested. If a trainer doesn't know an answer to your question, he or she should be able to direct you to the right sources of information.

Look for a trainer who is able to assist you with your special needs. A personal trainer should always have you fill out a health history questionnaire to determine your needs or limitations. If you have a medical condition or a past injury, a personal trainer should design a session that takes these into account. If you're under a doctor's care, the trainer should discuss any exercise concerns with your doctor and should ask for a health screening or release from your doctor. A quality trainer should assess and reassess your progress periodically.

How to Be a Good Client

A good client shows up on time, treats the trainer as a professional and is willing to learn. The client should prioritize the appointment along with other important items on the schedule for the day. A good client will focus on the exercise session and both the short- and long-term goals of the program. Reasonable rates for personal training vary widely, but a general guideline is between $25 and $100 per hour depending on whether the training takes place in a club or in your home.

counting the cost

One question almost everyone asks is, How much physical activity is enough? One way to answer this question is to count the cost—in calories that is! Scientific evidence reveals that an energy expenditure of *1,000 to 2,000 calories per week*—about *150 to 300 calories per day*—provides most of the health benefits associated with physical activity.

Use the following chart to see how many calories you're burning with physical activity. Multiply the number of minutes you spend in a physical activity by the calories burned per minute and add up the totals. If your activity is not on the list, find one on the list that seems to be about the same intensity and use that calorie level. If it's helpful for you, make several copies of the monitoring form so you can keep track of your activity and the number of calories you burn.

Activity	Calories Burned		
	Per Minute	In 30 Minutes	In One Hour
Brisk walking (15 to 20 minutes per mile)	5	150	300
Gardening (digging, planting, weeding)	5	150	300
Golf (walking)	5	150	300
Home repair (painting, carpentry)	5	150	300
Housework (mopping, washing windows)	5	150	300
Playing with children (running, roughhousing)	5	150	300
Water aerobics	5	150	300
Bicycling (leisurely—10 mph)	6	180	360
Dancing (folk, square, rock)	6	180	360
Yard work (shoveling, mowing, raking)	6	180	360
Weight training and calisthenics	6	180	360
Aerobic dance	7	210	420
Hiking	7	210	420
Ice-skating	7	210	420
Step aerobics	7	210	420
Tennis (doubles)	7	210	420
In-line skating	8	240	480
Power walking	8	240	480
Racquetball and squash	8	240	480
Stair-climbing machine	8	240	480
Tennis (singles)	8	240	480
Rowing machine	9	270	540
Bicycling (12 mph)	9	270	540
Ski machine	9	270	540
Swimming (moderate effort)	9	270	540
Basketball	10	300	600
Jogging (12 minutes per mile)	10	300	600
Jumping rope	10	300	600
Walking up stairs	10	300	600
Running (10 minutes per mile)	14	420	840

Activity Chart

Day/Date

Activity	Minutes	Calories per Minute	Total Calories
Daily Totals			

exercising outdoors

One of the best ways to get active is to get out and enjoy God's beautiful creation. There are many enjoyable and beneficial activities you can do outdoors, such as walking, hiking, bicycling, swimming and other recreational sports. However, when it comes to exercising outdoors, there are several things you can do to increase the enjoyment and safety of the activities you choose. It's important to consider weather, clothing, equipment and environment when exercising outdoors. Also, some activities such as downhill skiing, in-line skating and bicycling are more risky and require more precautions for safety. Choose activities you enjoy, but *take it slow and play it smart!*

Tips for Exercising Safely Outdoors

When exercising outdoors, there are several things you need to keep in mind to prevent injury or illness.

What to Wear

A good pair of shoes is the most important piece of equipment for exercising outdoors. Here are some tips for selecting a pair of exercise shoes.

- The best shoe is the one that fits your foot well, not necessarily the most expensive. Try on several pairs before buying. Does the shoe feel natural when you walk? Keep trying until you find one that feels right!
- Make sure the shoe supports your arch and has plenty of room for your toes; allow for a thumb's width between your toes and the end of the shoe. Keep your toenails trimmed!
- For walking or jogging, choose a flexible shoe with good cushioning. Don't go hiking in tennis shoes; wear the appropriate boot or shoe.
- For court and field sports, consider a high-top shoe to protect your ankles.
- Wear cotton or nylon athletic socks. It's not necessary to wear a double layer of socks.

When deciding what clothing to wear, consider the weather and light conditions.

- Whether exercising in the heat or cold, always wear clothing that can be layered and easily removed or put back on as your body temperature changes.
- Check with a local sports store for the best clothing and protective gear for your activity.
- Wear reflective and light-colored clothing, and carry a flashlight at dusk or at night.
- Consider carrying a small backpack or fanny pack to store extra clothing.
- When exercising in the heat, avoid clothing that does not ventilate well, such as rubberized suits or sweatsuits. Wearing such clothing is a dangerous practice that can lead to dehydration and heat stroke!

Weather

Extreme temperatures affect how your body responds to exercise. High temperatures and humidity or cold temperatures and wind place additional stress on your body. Check the weather forecast before heading outdoors. *Always decrease your intensity level and take it slow when it's very hot or cold!*

Tips for Beating the Heat

- It's a hot day when the temperature is above 85 degrees or when the temperature plus the humidity is greater than 130 (i.e., 80 degrees + 55% humidity = 135).
- It takes 10 to 14 days to adapt to the heat. If you're exercising in hot conditions, cut your intensity and duration in half and gradually increase your activity as your body adapts to the heat.
- Drink water before, during and after exercise. Drink at least five to eight ounces of cool water 15 minutes before and then every 15 to 20 minutes during exercise.
- On really hot days, exercise during the coolest part of the day or exercise indoors.
- Wear lightweight, loose-fitting clothes, a hat and sunscreen to protect you from the sun. If you wear a hat, make sure it allows for ventilation.

Tips for Exercising Safely in the Cold

- Don't just rely on the thermometer; the windchill greatly increases the risk of exercising in the cold.
- Dress warmly and in layers that can be easily removed. Several layers warm better than one heavy jacket. Because physical activity quickly generates body heat, it's important to be able to remove layers as your body heats up.
- Wool and synthetic fabrics are good choices because they whisk moisture away from your body. Wear an outer layer that keeps out the wind and moisture.
- Much of your body's heat can be lost through your head and neck, so wear a hat and scarf. Don't forget to protect your hands too.
- Watch out for slick surfaces caused by rain and snow.
- It's just as important to drink water in the cold as in the heat.
- When exercising in the cold, stay close to home or other shelter.

A Note About Altitude

Altitude increases the stress of physical activity. It's harder for your body to take in oxygen above 5,000 feet. This means your heart, lungs and muscles have to work harder. Symptoms of altitude sickness include lightheadedness, dizziness, nausea and unusual shortness of breath. Give yourself a couple of days to get use to the higher elevation, and cut back the intensity of your activities.

fitting in strength training

Strong muscles and bones are important for good health and an active life. While some loss of strength is a part of aging, most people lose strength because they don't get enough physical activity. To ensure that you have the energy, independence and mobility you need for a full and productive life, it's important to include some strength training in your physical activity program.

Studies find that strength training results in several important health benefits. Here's how the health and fitness benefits of strength training compare to aerobic exercise.

Health and Fitness Component	Strength Training	Aerobic Exercise
Increases ability to work and play	+ + +	+ + +
Improves balance in old age	+ + +	+ + +
Lowers blood pressure	+	+ +
Improves blood sugar	+ +	+ + +
Lowers body fat	+ + +	+ + +
Increases bone density	+ + +	+ +
Improves blood cholesterol levels	+	+ +
Increases strength	+ + +	+
Increases metabolic rate	+ +	+ +
Increases muscle mass	+ + +	+ +

+ Some benefit   + + Strong benefit   + + + Very strong benefit

Regular strength training gives you a new awareness of your body, makes you feel more firm and toned, increases metabolism and enhances quality of life by promoting mobility, maintaining strength and reducing risk of chronic disease.

Studies show that muscles and bones never lose their responsiveness to strength training; strength gains of nearly 200 percent have been achieved in 80- and 90-year-old men and women.

A study reported in the *Journal of the American Medical Association* found that women over age 50 significantly increased their muscle strength and bone density with regular weight training twice a week. The women in this study increased their strength by 75 percent and their bone density by 1 percent. The women who did no strength training lost strength, muscle mass and bone density.

A study in the elderly found that 12 weeks of resistance training increased daily energy expenditure by 15 percent.

Beginning a Strength-Training Program

Strength training does not require a lot of equipment or a health-club membership. Strength training can be done at home, in the office or just about anywhere!

Experts recommend that you include strength training in your activity routine two to three times each week. The goal is to find a resistance you can lift between 8 to 15 times without straining. Include at least one exercise for each of the major muscles: shoulders, back, chest, arms, stomach and legs.

Choosing Equipment

You can increase your strength simply by using your own body weight. No equipment is needed! Exercises that don't require special equipment include crunches (a type of sit-up), deep knee bends and push-ups. Add handheld weights, ankle weights or elastic exercise bands, and you have all you need for a complete program at home, at work or on the road.

Getting Started

- Whether you choose to use weight machines, handheld weights, elastic bands or your own body weight, the method for training remains the same.
- You only need to do strength exercises two or three days each week.
- When first starting, you only need to do each exercise one time or one set.

- Choose a resistance you can do 8 to 15 times without straining too hard or fatiguing the muscle completely. When first starting a strength-training program, it's best to start with very light resistance.
- Don't hold your breath and don't strain. Breathe easily throughout the exercise.
- Do some stretching and light activity to warm-up before starting and to cool down when finished.

Exercises to Get You Started

- **Deep Knee Bends**—Stand in front of a sturdy chair. The seat should be higher than the level of your knees. Keeping your back straight, bend at the knees and hips as if you were going to sit down. As your rear touches the chair's edge, slowly stand back up. If this is too difficult, start by sitting in the chair with your rear scooted toward the front. From this sitting position, stand up. Push off with your hands if you need to. Sit down normally and repeat.
- **Push-Ups**—Lie on your stomach, placing your hands shoulder-width apart at chest level. Keeping your back straight and both knees on the floor, push your body away from the floor in one smooth motion. Once your arms are straight, lower yourself back down. As you get stronger, do the push-ups while lifting your knees off the ground too. For an easier version, do the push-up leaning against the wall. Slowly bend at the elbows, allowing your chest to move toward the wall. Push your body away from the wall in one smooth motion.
- **Crunches**—Lie on your back with knees bent at a 90-degree angle and feet flat on the floor. Cross your hands over your chest or rest them on your legs. Slowly lift and curl your upper back and shoulder blades off the floor. You only need to lift your shoulders a few inches off the floor. You should feel some tightness in your stomach. Slowly curl back down.
- **Arm Curls**—Stand or sit with your arms hanging at your side and palms facing away from your body. Working only one arm at a time, keep your elbows close to your side as you slowly lift a handheld weight or elastic band (stand on the opposite end of the band or tie it to a table leg) by curling the weight up to your shoulder. Lower and repeat. Repeat with the opposite arm.

How to Progress

When 8 to 15 repetitions of any given exercise become easy, you may be ready to progress to the next level. Here are some ideas for the next step.

- Add a few more repetitions.
- Increase the weight or resistance.
- Repeat the exercise twice or even three times as your strength increases.
- Learn new exercises.

a flexible fitness program

Stretching is a simple and relaxing activity that offers a variety of important health and fitness benefits. A regular program of stretching exercises gives you increased flexibility in your muscles and joints, which helps you feel more relaxed, prevents injury and improves your ease of movement. Stretching also prevents the loss of flexibility and the pain and stiffness that make doing even simple activities difficult later in life. Unfortunately, flexibility is the most often overlooked part of an activity program.

Are You Flexible Enough?

- Are your muscles and joints sore and stiff after yard work, exercise or recreational activities?
- Are you sore and stiff first thing in the morning?
- Do you feel less agile and flexible than you did a few years ago?
- Does your range of motion seem limited when doing certain activities?

If you answered yes to any of these questions, you'll probably benefit from a program of regular stretching. Remember that flexibility is important for overall health and well-being, too.

The Best Time to Stretch

Stretching should be done as part of your warm-up before and cooldown after physical activity. You may also want to do a routine program of stretching several times each week. In fact, stretching can be done any time.

Guidelines for Safe Stretching

- Before stretching, warm up your body with 3 to 5 minutes of light activity.
- All stretches should be performed slowly and smoothly. Never bounce or jerk.
- Focus on the muscles and joints you're stretching and keep your body relaxed.
- Stretch to the point that you feel mild muscle tension. Don't stretch to the point of pain! Overstretching will do more harm than good.
- Hold each stretch for 15 to 20 seconds. Relax and breathe easily during each stretch. Never hold your breath.
- Avoid stretches that cause you to arch your back or neck backward or put stress on your knees.
- Don't do any stretch that could cause you to lose your balance and fall.
- Never compare yourself to others. Flexibility is not about how far you can stretch; it's about loosening and relaxing the muscles and joints.

Exercises

The following exercises are basic stretches for the major muscles and joints. Spend more time on your stiffest areas, but try to do all these stretches several times each week. You can do all the stretches at one time or do different stretches at different times of the day. The best way is to start with your neck and work your way down. Repeat each of the following stretches two to three times. Remember to relax, go slow and enjoy the time you spend stretching. Stretching is a great time to pray and meditate on Scripture.

Neck

These can be done sitting or standing.
- While looking straight ahead, tilt your head to the side as though you're trying to touch your ear to your shoulder. Hold the stretch for a few seconds; then repeat the movement to the other side.
- Next, try to touch your chin to your chest. Go down only as far as is comfortable, hold for a few seconds and take a deep breath. Return to the starting position.

Shoulders and Arms

These can be done sitting or standing.
- Reach up and over your head with one or both arms, as if trying to touch the ceiling. Bend slightly to each side. Repeat with the other arm.
- Next, reach forward with one arm and then stretch it across your chest toward the opposite shoulder. Increase the stretch by pulling with the opposite arm. Repeat with the other arm.

- Starting with your arms at your side, shrug your shoulders by bringing them up toward your ears. Lower your shoulders while stretching them backward, pulling the shoulder blades together. Return to the starting position with your arms at your sides.
- Hold your arms straight out to the side. Make wide circles with your arms, both forward and backward, by turning them at the shoulder. Make circles with your wrists, too.

Trunk and Sides

- With your arms at your side and feet at least shoulder width apart, bend toward one side while sliding your arm down the side of your hip and leg. Stretch only as far as is comfortable and watch your balance. Keep your back and neck straight while doing this stretch. Repeat, this time stretching toward the other side.

Lower Back

- While sitting in a chair with your knees bent, bend forward from the waist and slide your hands down your legs toward your toes. Bend down only as far as is comfortable. Hold the stretch for a few seconds and rise back up slowly.
- Lie on your back with your knees bent and feet flat on the ground. Use your hands to pull one knee up toward the chest, while keeping your leg bent. As you pull up, press your back gently toward the floor. Keep the opposite leg bent at a 90-degree angle and your foot flat on the floor. Hold the stretch for a few seconds. Repeat with the other leg.
- Lie with your knees bent at a 90-degree angle and feet flat on the floor. Press the small of your back toward the floor while tightening your stomach muscles. Hold the stretch for a few seconds.
- Kneel on your hands and knees and relax your neck. Arch your back up like a cat, feeling the stretch across your back. Hold for a few seconds. Repeat.

Legs and Ankles

- Sit on the floor. With your legs extended and your knees slightly bent, stretch forward at the waist and try to touch your toes. You don't have to touch your toes—just bend forward until you feel a stretch in the back of your legs. Keep your head and back as straight as possible and breathe easily.
- Face a wall with your arms extended straight out in front of you. Move one foot forward and leave the other foot back one to two feet. Keeping the heel of your back foot on the ground and toes pointing forward, lean your body

toward the wall until you feel a mild stretch in your calf and heel. Hold the stretch for a few seconds. Repeat the stretch by changing the position of your feet.

- To loosen up ankle muscles, draw an imaginary circle with your foot by turning your foot at the ankle. Do circles in both directions. Repeat several times with each foot.

group exercise for fun and fitness

Group exercise simply refers to a group of people exercising together under the direction of an instructor. Often the exercises are set to music. The instructor, group members and music all work together to create a fun and beneficial workout. Group exercise classes are offered at fitness clubs, community centers and some workplaces. You can even do group exercise at home with special video. If you want, find a qualified instructor and get your own group together in the neighborhood, at church or at work.

Here's a list of some of the most popular group classes. Which ones do you enjoy?

☐ Aerobic dance (low/high-impact)
☐ Indoor cycling
☐ Jazzercise
☐ Boxing-type workouts
☐ Stepping (low/high impact)

☐ Group calisthenics/flexibility
☐ Water aerobics
☐ Combination of various types
☐ Circuit weight training
☐ Other: _____

The Benefits of Group Exercise

Check out the following benefits of group exercise. If several of these benefits sound important to you, group exercise may be a good choice.

- It's more fun to exercise with others.
- A well-trained instructor can provide motivation and education.
- The group can be a source of accountability.
- Provides variety for your physical activity routine.
- The music and environment make exercise more enjoyable.
- Can provide a total body workout: aerobics, strength building and stretching.

First Steps

Choosing the Right Instructor

Look for a nationally certified instructor who has the experience and knowledge to provide you with a safe, effective and enjoyable workout. A good instructor will learn your name, make eye contact during the session and put your workout before his or her own. The instructor should have you take your heart rate or teach you how to rate your intensity level. A good teacher will explain the benefits of each exercise, demonstrate how to do the exercise and modify movements for all skill and fitness levels.

Clothing and Shoes

Usually you don't need any special clothing. Choose clothing that allows you to move freely. It's important that the clothes you choose breathe, allowing sweat to evaporate. Avoid rubber suits and sweatshirts that don't absorb or pull moisture away from the skin. Most important, wear clothing that is comfortable—put fitness ahead of fashion! For dance or step classes, choose an aerobic shoe with good cushioning. Good heel and arch support is important. The shoe should be flexible, provide a broad base of support and have plenty of room for your toes. Running or walking shoes are not a good choice because they don't provide the support you need for side-to-side movements. A high-top shoe might provide more ankle support. Shop for shoes carefully.

Precautions

Before you reserve your spot in a group class, you need to take a few precautions.

- ***If you are a man over 40 or a woman over 50, or if you have underlying health problems, check with your doctor before participating in a vigorous exercise class.***
- Some aerobic dance and step classes are *high* impact (i.e., a lot of hopping, jumping and jogging). If you're just starting out or you have knee, ankle or back problems, choose classes that are *low* impact. Some classes can also be difficult if you have poor balance or coordination. Water aerobics might be a better choice.
- The skill and fitness levels needed for various classes differ. Choose a class that's best for you. The class should not fatigue or exhaust you. If you initially find the class difficult to follow, focus on learning the movements before worrying about intensity. Avoid exercising at a higher level of intensity than your body is used to; it's easy to overexert yourself trying to keep up with the class. If you have a hard time keeping up, slow down and take a break when necessary. Remember, you're doing this for your own health and fitness—not to compete with others.
- Learning to maintain proper body alignment and technique helps prevent injuries. Maintain good posture with shoulders back, chest lifted, back straight and pelvis tucked under. Try to stay relaxed and breathe easily. Avoid any movements that are uncomfortable for you or seem to put stress on your joints. Just because an instructor does a movement doesn't mean it's right for you. Talk to your instructor about other movements or stretches you can do instead. Using hand weights can increase the risk of injury in aerobic dance and stepping classes. In stepping classes avoid using benches that are too high—start with a 4- to 6-inch bench and work your way up as your fitness improves.
- Drink plenty of water. Drink at least 8 ounces of water 15 minutes before class and continue to drink water every 15 to 20 minutes during class. It's a good idea to keep a water bottle nearby while you exercise.

Components of a Group Exercise Class

Most classes consist of four or five phases. Each phase has an important purpose for both fitness and safety. These same phases should be a part of any exercise or physical activity you do.

- **Warm-Up Phase**—This prepares the body for more vigorous activity by allowing muscles and joints to loosen up and the heart and lungs to gradually begin delivering more blood and oxygen to the muscles. The warm-up should consist of at least 5 to 10 minutes of light activity and stretching.

- **Aerobic Phase**—This consists of continuous and rhythmic movement designed to improve health and cardiovascular endurance. The aerobic phase should not feel hard and should last 20 to 30 minutes. If the pace is uncomfortable or you're breathing so hard you can't carry on a conversation, *slow down!*

- **Transition Phase**—This short phase of light activity is important when you move from the aerobics phase to the calisthenics and flexibility phase.

- **Calisthenics and Flexibility Phase**—This consists of strengthening and stretching exercises to condition and tone the muscles, improve range of motion and lower the risk of injury.

- **Cooldown Phase**—This allows time for the body to safely transition back to normal activity. It's very important not to stop abruptly following moderate to vigorous activity. The cooldown should consist of at least 5 to 10 minutes of light activity and stretching.

home fitness equipment

Do you just not have time to make it to the fitness center? Do you feel uncomfortable working out in front of others? Maybe you don't have a fitness center nearby. Is a fitness center membership more than you're willing or able to pay? Maybe you would just like to have a backup for those days when you can't make it to the gym. Fortunately, you don't have to join a fitness center to get the benefits of physical activity. There are many great ways to fit physical activity into your life. Choose activities that you enjoy and can fit into your lifestyle. With a little planning, you can get all the physical activity you need in the comfort and convenience of your own home.

The Advantages of Home Exercise
- **Convenience**—No travel time and no special hours are required, and you don't have to worry about what to wear.
- **Privacy**—You can work out in the comfort of your own home and at your own speed, with no overcrowding.
- **Cost**—Depending on what activity and equipment you choose, exercising at home can be very economical.

The Disadvantages of Home Exercise
- **Less Variety**—A fitness center offers a greater variety of exercise and equipment options.
- **Self-Discipline**—Some people have a hard time motivating themselves to work out alone.
- **Distractions**—The television, telephone, spouse, kids and household chores may compete for your time and attention.
- **Cost**—Some fitness equipment may cost as much or more than a club membership.

Types of Equipment
There is no best exercise or piece of exercise equipment. The best one is the one that is right for you. Any activity that requires you to use your muscles or causes you to breathe a little harder is good for your body. Walking, jogging, bicycling, dancing and strength training are good examples. Choose the one you like best and do it regularly.

All of the following types of exercise equipment are good choices:

- Treadmills
- Skiing machines
- Elastic exercise bands
- Stationary or regular bicycles
- Rowers
- Stair climbers
- Strength equipment
- Jump ropes
- Aerobic or step videos
- Roller blades or skates

Don't just buy a piece of exercise equipment because you think it will be good for you. Here are some things to ask yourself before you buy.

- *What do I enjoy doing?*
- *Will I really enjoy working out at home? Why?*
- *Will I use the equipment regularly? Will I quickly get bored with it?* (Far too common is the exercise machine that becomes an expensive clothes rack or ends up in a garage sale or thrift shop!)
- *Have I used or bought home-exercise equipment before? What did I like about it? What did I dislike about it?*
- *Do I have a convenient place to put it?*
- *How much can I afford to spend?* (Set a budget before you go shopping.)

Selection Tips

When shopping for exercise equipment, look for something that gives you the feel of the activity you enjoy. You need to test equipment before you buy it. Does it seem to be well made? Does it feel solid and durable? Give the equipment a good test ride—five minutes is not enough!

Stationary Bikes—Low Impact and Space Saving

- Choose a bike with a smooth pedaling motion.
- Make sure you're comfortable with the pedaling resistance and that it's easily adjusted.
- A comfortable, adjustable-tilt seat is a must. If bicycle seats are typically uncomfortable for you, look for a recumbent bike which allows you to sit in a padded chair with your legs extended in front of you.
- Some bikes have arm levers that allow you to work your upper body, too.

Treadmills—All-Season Walking and Jogging

- You'll need plenty of room—both in length and width—to comfortably walk or jog.
- The walking or jogging surface should be stable and provide good shock absorption (i.e., doesn't bounce or rock back and forth).
- Choose a machine with handrails for balance and a control panel that is easy to reach and use. It's best if you can adjust the speed and elevation while exercising.
- Strong motors ($1\frac{1}{4}$ to $1\frac{3}{4}$ horsepower) make for a quieter and longer-lasting treadmill.

Stair-Climbing Machines—Low Impact and Space Saving

- Choose a sturdy machine with good stability.
- Look for independent steps that have a smooth motion; chain or cable systems are generally smoother than hydraulic (air-powered) systems.
- It should allow for variable resistance (i.e., you set the tension, or workload).
- Make sure it is equipped with comfortable handrails.

Cross-Country Skiing and Rowing Machines—Variable Resistance

- Look for a machine that works both the upper and lower body.
- Look for stability; the machine shouldn't rock back and forth.
- The machine should provide smooth sliding motion of skis, with seat and arm pulleys.
- Make sure it allows for variable resistance (i.e., you set the tension, or workload).

Weights—Strengthen Muscles and Increase Bone Density

- **Complex Systems**—Multistation resistance machines certainly have their place, but they are not affordable or practical for everyone.
- **Simple Systems**—You can get all the strength training you need with handheld weights, elastic exercise bands, dumbbells and an exercise mat or bench.

Additional Tips

- If you know someone with home exercise equipment, ask to try it out before buying your own.
- Analyze your workout room. The area you plan to exercise in should be spacious and pleasant with good lighting and ventilation. Some people like to read or watch television while using their exercise equipment.

- Because you must test the equipment extensively before you purchase it, wear your workout gear when shopping!
- Buy from a knowledgeable retailer. Discuss warranties, installation, maintenance and service plans.
- Check out used equipment for purchase.

join the club

Tips for Selecting a Fitness Center

Are you looking for the best way to fit physical activity into your life? There is no *one* best way. The best way is the one that works for you. Joining a fitness center can be a great choice for some people. Fitness centers offer a wide selection of equipment and activities to help you achieve and maintain a physically active lifestyle and all the benefits that go along with it. They also provide a safe and comfortable environment in all kinds of weather, almost any time of the day.

Is Joining a Fitness Center Right for Me?

You have several options when it comes to fitting physical activity into your life. You can purchase home exercise equipment, exercise outdoors, walk in the mall or fit *lifestyle* physical activities into your daily routine (i.e., taking the stairs instead of the elevator, working in your yard, etc.). The most important thing is to choose activities that you enjoy and that fit into your lifestyle. Before joining a fitness center, ask yourself the following questions:

- *Have I been a member of a fitness center before?*
- *(If yes.) Did I enjoy and use it regularly?*
- *Can I afford all the fees* (initiation, membership and classes)?
- *Is there a fitness center close to my home or work?*
- *Do I have the time to use a fitness center regularly?*
- *Do I enjoy working out with others?*
- *Do I enjoy having a wide variety of exercise options from which to choose?*
- *Will I benefit from having an expert staff of fitness professionals to help me choose and maintain an effective, safe physical-activity program?*

- *Will joining a fitness center provide the motivation and inspiration I need to get and stay active?*
- *What specific benefits* (i.e., equipment, group classes, supervision or amenities) *am I looking for from a fitness center?*

How Do I Choose a Fitness Center That's Right for Me?

When selecting a fitness center, there are several important things to consider.

- **Is it convenient?** Studies show that you are more likely to use a center if it's within 10 to 12 minutes of your home or workplace. Remember, lack of time and inconvenient location are two common reasons people give for dropping out of a fitness program!
- **Does it provide a safe, friendly and comfortable environment?** Ask the club to allow you to work out for several days before joining— many clubs will. This helps you to see if you are comfortable in the club and enables you to become familiar with the equipment, staff and other members. If a club won't allow you a trial period, look elsewhere!
- **Is the staff trained and certified in exercise instruction and counseling?** Among the top certifications are the American College of Sports Medicine, the American Counsel on Exercise, the National Strength and Conditioning Association and the Cooper Institute.
- **Does it offer classes for all levels of fitness and skill?** Make sure the club has classes at your level at times convenient for you.
- **Does the center have a wide selection of exercise equipment?** Is the equipment clean and in good working order? Check for "out of order" signs. Check the size of the crowd at the time you will be using the facility and the availability of the equipment you'll want to use.

- **What extra features are you looking for?** Do you want a swimming pool, racquet courts, locker rooms, private showers, massage services, steam rooms, hot tubs or cafeteria?
- **How much are you willing to spend on a membership?** Do you want to pay monthly or annually?
- **What special programs and services does the club offer?** Are child care, educational programs, nutritional counseling, personal training, etc. available? Are these important to you?

Things to Look For

- **Does the club have high-pressure sales techniques?** You need to have time to think about your decision and review the contract and terms of membership. If you feel pressured, that club's probably not for you!
- **Does the center offer only (or pressure you to sign) long-term contracts (i.e., longer than one year)?** You may prefer a monthly membership at first to see if the fitness center is right for you.
- **Are the membership options and contracts hard to understand?** Contracts should be easy to understand, and options should be easy to choose from.
- **Does the fitness center representative ask you about your health and medical history?** Knowing your history is important for designing a fitness program that is right for you.
- **Does the fitness center appear to be understaffed?** You should have readily available help when you need it while working out.

Tips for Getting the Most Out of a Fitness Center

- Ask the staff to give you an orientation to the center and the equipment. Staff should always be available to answer your questions and help you use the equipment safely and effectively.
- Choose a work-out time that's convenient for you. Schedule your exercise time just as you would any other important appointment.
- Choose activities and equipment you enjoy.
- Set specific goals for health and physical activity to keep you motivated.
- Get a loved one, coworker or friend to join you. The support of a buddy often keeps you on track.
- You may need to ask for help around the house or at work so that you can fit in your workout.

overcoming obstacles to physical activity

Most of us don't need to be told that physical activity is good for us. While knowing why and how to become more physically active is important, the more important question is, *How can I get started and then stick with it?* Have you been physically active in the past and then stopped? You're not alone; more than 50 percent of people who start an exercise program drop out within the first three to six months. By the end of a year only one out of four are still active. There are many reasons people give for not starting or sticking with a physical activity program. By making yourself aware of your personal obstacles to physical activity, you can improve your chances of sticking with your program for a lifetime.

See if you recognize yourself in the following list of excuses, and then read the helpful solutions:

I Don't Enjoy Exercise

Don't exercise. Find physical activities you enjoy—try a sport or active hobby. Find someone to exercise with you. Listen to music, pray or find other ways to take your mind off the activity.

I Don't Have Time for Exercise

You have to make time—30 minutes several days a week is all it takes. Break up your activity into shorter segments of 5, 10 or 15 minutes. Schedule activity just like you would any other important meeting. Ask family and friends to help you make the time.

I'm Too Tired to Exercise

Low energy levels are often the result of low fitness and too much stress; regular physical activity improves fitness, increases energy levels and is a great stress reliever.

Exercise Is Not Convenient

Physical activity can be done anywhere and anytime. Look for opportunities to fit physical activity into your day—walk during your lunch break, buy home exercise equipment, find a health club nearby. Community centers, YMCAs, colleges and some churches have fitness facilities that are convenient and affordable.

Exercise Is Too Hard

Activity doesn't have to be hard to be beneficial. The important thing is that you choose activities you enjoy. Many people want quick results, so they start off doing too much too soon.

I Don't Have Anyone to Exercise with Me

Maybe you're not asking enough people; ask family, friends, neighbors, coworkers and church acquaintances. Join a sports or recreation group. Check with community centers, colleges and local fitness clubs.

I Don't Feel Any Different When I Exercise

Don't expect to feel good right away. It takes time for your body to adapt to regular physical activity. After four to six weeks of regular activity, you should start feeling and seeing a difference. Monitor your progress along the way.

I'm Too Overweight and Out of Shape

Physical activity and good health have nothing to do with the way you look or how well you perform; it's about being the best you can be. Never compare yourself to others. Always remember that you're truly fearfully and wonderfully made (see Psalm 139:14)! Choose activities you enjoy and do them in a comfortable environment. Don't let your feelings about yourself or your perceptions about what other people think keep you from achieving your goals.

I Don't Have Any Reason to Be Active

Find reasons! Prayerfully consider the benefits of living a more physically active lifestyle—reduced risk of heart disease, cancer, diabetes, high blood pressure and osteoporosis; more energy; weight loss and maintenance; improved mood; higher quality of life. The stronger your motivations, the more likely you'll be successful. Read Mark 12:28-31; Psalm 139:14 and 1 Corinthians 6:19-20. How do these verses speak of the importance of taking good care of yourself? When we are physically fit, we can better serve the Lord.

The Weather Is Bad

Get out of the habit of using weather as an excuse for not being physically active. With the appropriate clothing and gear, you can enjoy activity all year long. If you can't get outside, work out in your home, walk in the mall or join a fitness center.

My Family and Friends Are Not Supportive

Family and friends who aren't supportive can make it very difficult. The key is communication. Find creative ways to get others involved in your program. Surround yourself with others who are more supportive. Be sensitive to others, but don't allow them to sabotage your efforts. Get out there and do it anyway, and maybe when they see the benefits, they'll be motivated to join you!

Exercise Seems So Self-Centered

You are God's good creation and your body is the temple of the Holy Spirit. You're responsible for caring for your body. A physically active lifestyle and the benefits it brings will give you the energy you need for effective living and serving others. The focus of your activity should be on caring for your body and honoring God.

What are *your* obstacles? You need to anticipate that you will have difficulties. Things will interfere with your ability and desire to exercise. The key is to expect the obstacles, plan ahead and make a commitment to stick with your goals.

What is keeping you from being active now? What obstacles are most likely to interfere with your physical activity program? How can you get back on track if you stop? Make sure your obstacles are not just excuses. We find the time and the ways to do the things that are important to us. Learn to turn negative thinking into positive: *I can, I will, I'm willing to try*.

putting your best foot forward

In the past, you may have given little thought to the kind of athletic shoes you buy; but if you're going to be serious about a physically active lifestyle, you need to be serious about your feet. Your foot contains 26 bones and has to bear more than six times your body weight during running and jumping activities! A bad pair of shoes can lead to problems as minor as blisters and as major as knee problems.

Selecting the Right Shoe

It's important to select the right shoes for your activity. Runners were the first to buy into the idea of specialty shoes. Today experts suggest that people purchase shoes that complement the sport for which they were designed, which means that a person may want several pairs. The following are commonly used:

- **Running**—These are considered forward-motion shoes. They're lightweight, have good cushioning and a raised toe that enables the shoe to roll forward.
- **Walking**—Slightly heavier than some other athletic shoes, they often have features called "roll bars" or "footbridges" that give added support for people who *overpronate* (see definition in next section).
- **Tennis**—These shoes are flatter underneath than a running shoe and, therefore, have more support and stability when moving in a side-to-side, or lateral, motion. A leather upper gives additional support.
- **Basketball**—Similar to tennis shoes, they have more ankle support and more cushioning for jumping.
- **Cross-trainers**—They're much heavier than running shoes and don't have as much support. They work well for people who enjoy several different activities, but they're not recommended for any one particular sport.

In addition, there are specialty shoes for biking, soccer, hiking and other activities. Seek the advice of someone who really knows your sport before making a purchase.

Checking Your Gait

When walking or running, few of us have a neutral gait. Many people roll too far to the inside of the foot, which is called *overpronating*. Others *underpronate* (supinate), meaning that they don't roll enough to the inside. Both gaits can be hard on your feet, knees, hips and back if you have the wrong pair of shoes. Fortunately, a well-fitting shoe can often correct these problems.

What Type of Foot Pattern Do You Have?

Step out of the shower with wet feet and walk across a dry floor. Can you see your entire footprint? If so, you may have a flattened arch and a tendency to overpronate. If you see an island of the forefoot and an island of the heel with dry space between, you probably have a higher arch and a tendency to under-pronate. A person who overpronates needs a stiff shoe, whereas someone who underpronates needs a flexible one.

Making a Purchase

When Is It Time for a New Pair?

When to replace shoes depends on how active you are. As a general rule, experts recommend replacing running shoes every 350 to 500 miles. The runner who is heavy and strikes the foot hard against the pavement should replace a shoe closer to the 350-mile range. With a lot of use, you can lose about 60 percent of the cushioning in six months; even if the shoes don't show major wear, remember that they can quickly lose their shock-absorption capacity and some of their stability. If you start noticing a new ache or pain, it may be time for a new pair of shoes!

Walkers don't need to replace their shoes as often—usually after about 600 miles of use.

Take Your Old Pair with You

Surprisingly, experts say that about 80 percent of the people are wearing shoes that are too short. It makes sense to take your old pair with you when you shop and to go late in the day when your feet have expanded. Ask a knowledgeable salesperson to evaluate your old shoes, which will help them steer you to the best models. You may want to go to a specialty shop instead of a discount outlet. A good salesperson can look at your shoe and observe several patterns. For example:

- **What do the soles look like?** Where has wear occurred? Many people wear out the outside corner (the point of first contact of the shoe with the ground). Wearing out the inside corner may be a sign of overpronation, which increases your risk of injury if the shoe is not right.
- **What is the shoe's design?** Is the shoe right for the activity you do? Is the shoe comfortable? How does the shoe fit? Is it a special size?

Selecting a Brand

There is no one best shoe or brand. Never buy a particular brand or type of shoe just because it works for someone you know. The best shoe is the one that fits your foot. There are several major brands of shoes; most contain the same kinds of rubber, nylon, leather, etc. However, shoes vary from one manufacturer to the next. Try on several pairs, and make your decision based on comfort rather than the brand name.

Buying Tips

- Make sure you have a thumbnail's width of space between your longest toe and the front of the shoe.
- Select shoes based on your weight and foot type. A 100-pound woman, for example, may need a lighter-weight pair of shoes than someone weighing 175 pounds.
- The shoe should be snug without pinching. Don't expect a pair of athletic shoes to fit as tightly as a dress shoe.
- Choose shoes that fit snugly without slipping on your heel.
- Lace up the shoes, and walk, run and jump around the store or outside. Remember: If the shoes aren't comfortable in the store, they won't fit well when you get home.
- Sizes vary, depending on the manufacturer. Be willing to try on several sizes until you find the one that fits and feels the best.
- If you find a shoe that works well for you, consider buying a second pair. Models are frequently discontinued. In addition, rotating two pairs helps extend the life of your shoes.
- Don't purchase an ill-fitting pair of shoes just because they're on sale. You may end up paying more in the long run in the form of shin splints, sore knees or other problems.

Allow for a Breaking-In Period

Of course, it goes without saying that you need to break in a new pair of shoes. Don't purchase running shoes and attempt to run a marathon the next day. Gradually increase the use of a new pair of shoes; it takes a little time for the shoe to form to your foot. By all means, however, use them regularly! With a good pair of shoes, you'll likely get more out of your workout—and your feet will thank you!

sports and recreational activities

There are many different ways to fit physical activity into your lifestyle. The first step is to find activities you enjoy. Then you need to get out there and do them on a regular basis. Sports and recreational activities can be a great way to fit in physical activity. Check out the following benefits:

- They strengthen muscles, burn calories and reduce stress just as well as other types of exercise.
- They provide opportunities to enjoy your health and fitness. Playing and having fun helps you stay young and keeps you motivated.
- They allow you to spend time with family and friends and meet new people too! Remember, relationships are just as important to your overall health and well-being as exercise and good nutrition.
- The competitive nature of some sports can inspire you to set fitness goals and stay motivated. Setting a goal such as finishing a 10K race or playing in a tennis league can make your workouts more meaningful.

Select Recreational Activities You Enjoy

No matter what your skill, coordination or fitness level, you can find activities that you can enjoy. Find one or two sports or recreational activities you enjoy, and fit them into your fitness routine one to three times each week. Consider the following list of possibilities:

Badminton	Golf	Skiing	Tennis
Basketball	Hiking	Soccer	Volleyball
Bike Rallies	Racquetball	Softball	
Fun runs/walks	Skating	Squash	

Individual Sports and Activities

- **Fun Runs/Walks**—Many people enjoy participating in local fun runs or walks. These community events offer challenge and camaraderie. Most people don't run to compete with others; their goal is to finish the race and feel good about their accomplishment. Training for a local event is a great way to keep you motivated and add variety to your exercise routine. Joining a walking or running group is a great way to meet other people with similar interests.

- **Bike Rallies**—If you enjoy bicycling, you might want to train for a bike rally. Bike rallies are generally anywhere from 25 to 100 miles long. Choose your distance and start training. Training for a rally is a great motivator. Participating in a rally provides a great source of accomplishment and is a fun way to meet other people. Well-organized rides attract thousands of riders of all fitness levels and create a fun and exciting environment. Most cities also have bicycle clubs that get together on the weekends for longer rides and fellowship. *Never do a longer event, whether walking, running or cycling, without proper training.*

- **Skating**—There are several ways to skate these days. The two most popular ways are in-line skating (i.e., roller-blading) and ice-skating. Actually, in-line skating is one of the fastest growing recreational activities in this country. Skating is a great aerobic exercise and a good way to burn calories. Skating does take a little more skill than walking, jogging or bicycling, and the risk of injury is much higher. Before making the investment, rent a pair of skates and take formal lessons. When in-line skating, wear wrist guards, protective padding and a helmet.

- **Skiing**—Many people have the opportunity to go downhill skiing one or more times each year. The annual ski trip can be a great motivator to keep yourself in shape. To ski enjoyably and safely you need a moderate to high level of cardiovascular endurance, muscular fitness, flexibility, balance and coordination. Spend at least two or three months getting yourself in condition to go skiing. The risk of injury during skiing is very high, and the injuries can be severe: broken bones and torn ligaments. High altitude and cold temperatures are also important safety considerations.

- **Golf**—This popular sport provides a great opportunity to enjoy the outdoors. Golf is more of a game of skill than it is of physical fitness. However, by walking and carrying your own clubs, golf can count toward your weekly physical activity goal. Physical fitness can improve your game. To be successful in golf, focus on three components of fitness: strength/power, flexibility and cardiovascular endurance. Cardiovascular endurance is essential to help keep your energy up during a long round of golf. Flexibility exercises increase your range of motion and prevent injury. Muscular fitness can improve the power and speed of your swing.

Racquet Sports

Racquet sports such as tennis, racquetball and squash are popular and can be played as singles or doubles. All of them offer a moderate to vigorous workout, depending on the intensity you put into it. Playing singles usually requires more effort and burns more calories. In addition to enjoying health and fitness benefits, you will also develop balance, agility and coordination. The more fit you are, the better you'll play. Develop a regular fitness routine to help improve your game and lower your risk of injury. You need cardiovascular endurance, flexibility and strength to play your best.

For equipment all you need to play is a good pair of shoes, a racquet (or just your hand for handball), a partner and a court. Shoes are probably your most important piece of equipment. You'll need a good court shoe with adequate cushioning. You'll also need good heel and ankle support because these sports have a lot of side-to-side movement. Many of the sports require protective eyewear. Check with a YMCA, local fitness club or recreation center to sign up for lessons, or find a local racquet club to help you improve your game and meet other people.

Team Sports

Team sports such as basketball, softball, volleyball and soccer have both fitness and social benefits. These sports can be light, moderate or vigorous in intensity depending on the sport and how hard you play. Regardless of the intensity, including team sports in your fitness program can offer a variety of benefits. Low-intensity sports such as softball and volleyball are a great outlet for competition and fellowship. Regardless of the sport you choose, the more fit you are, the better you'll play. You need cardiovascular endurance, muscular fitness and flexibility to play your best.

Be careful if you play team sports only sporadically. It's easy to let the competitive drive take over and overexert yourself—the weekend-warrior syndrome. Some sports can take a greater toll on your body, especially as you grow older. Make sure you wear the appropriate shoes and protective gear. As you would for any exercise, spend some time warming up with light activity and stretching before playing. Cool down gradually after playing vigorous sports such as basketball or soccer.

staying active while traveling

Almost everyone travels—whether it's for business, a weekend getaway or a family vacation. Many people find it more difficult to stay physically active while on the road. The good news is that with a little planning, you can enjoy the benefits of physical activity while traveling. Sure, it may be a little harder to make time for physical activity when you travel, but the benefits will be well worth the effort.

Business Trips

When traveling for business, sometimes it's hard to make your own schedule—schedules are tight, meetings run late, flights are delayed and colleagues often want to entertain you. The key to a physically active business trip is—you guessed it—planning! Try the following tips for fitting in activity when you travel on business:

- Rise a little earlier in the morning to fit in some activity; this way you can't miss it!
- Schedule activity into your day just like you schedule meetings.
- Make sure colleagues know that physical activity is important to you.
- When traveling, wear comfortable shoes or carry tennis shoes in your carry-on bag. Walk between meetings or while waiting for your flight—even 10 minutes of exercise will help.
- Fit in activity by taking the stairs instead of the elevator, carrying your own bags and walking wherever you can.

Vacations

Traveling for pleasure is a great way to enjoy your health and fitness: hike in the mountains, walk along a secluded beach, bicycle through the countryside or windsurf over the waves. Don't think so much about following your usual routine; look for new ways to be physically active. When you're planning your trip, take time to plan ways to fit activity into your schedule. Check out the following ideas for active travel:

- Local attractions such as parks, zoos, nature trails and other activities can provide opportunities to see the sights and get some activity at the same time!
- Planning ahead allows you to take clothing, shoes and equipment you will need for physical activity.
- Plan active vacations, such as hiking or camping. Stay at hotels with exercise facilities.
- Try to find ways to be active with your traveling companions: rent bicycles, skates or other recreational equipment. It's often easier to stay active if you have the support of others.
- Find out about the weather conditions before you go so that you can pack the right clothing.
- Take along recreational equipment such as racquets, golf clubs, a jump rope, etc.

Healthful Tips for Active Travelers

Check with the Hotel Where You Will Be Staying
- Does it provide an exercise room?
- Are there safe walking paths nearby?
- Is there a mall nearby where you can walk?
- Are there local fitness facilities you can use?
- Pack a swimsuit and take advantage of the hotel pool.

Be Prepared for Changes in Plans
- If the weather is bad, walk in a mall or go to an indoor fitness center.
- For a quick workout, take along elastic exercise bands, hand weights, a jump rope, music or an exercise video for activity in your hotel room.
- If a flight is delayed, take a brisk walk around the airport terminal.

You may need to lower your expectations when traveling—even 10 minutes of activity is beneficial. Don't skip activity just because you can't do your usual routine.

Doing your activity first thing in the morning is a great way to fit it in. This way if a meeting runs late, a flight is delayed or something else comes up, you've done your activity for the day.

Avoid overdoing it. You want to be rested and relaxed when you travel. Don't push yourself when you're tired. Sometimes rest will do you more good than exercise. Don't let trying to fit in a workout become another stress when you travel. There's plenty of time for physical activity when you get home.

While traveling, try to get plenty of sleep, drink lots of water and eat healthful foods. Carry healthy snacks with you when you travel. A little snack can give you the boost you need to make it to the next meal. If you get too hungry, you may opt for eating out rather than working out!